T0296230

Critical Care EEG Basics

Critical Care
EEG Basics

Rapid Bedside EEG Reading for Acute Care Providers

Neville M. Jadeja
University of Massachusetts Medical School

Kyle C. Rossi
University of Massachusetts Medical School

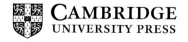
CAMBRIDGE
UNIVERSITY PRESS

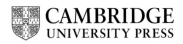

Shaftesbury Road, Cambridge CB2 8EA, United Kingdom

One Liberty Plaza, 20th Floor, New York, NY 10006, USA

477 Williamstown Road, Port Melbourne, VIC 3207, Australia

314–321, 3rd Floor, Plot 3, Splendor Forum, Jasola District Centre, New Delhi – 110025, India

103 Penang Road, #05-06/07, Visioncrest Commercial, Singapore 238467

Cambridge University Press is part of Cambridge University Press & Assessment, a department of the University of Cambridge.

We share the University's mission to contribute to society through the pursuit of education, learning and research at the highest international levels of excellence.

www.cambridge.org
Information on this title: www.cambridge.org/9781009261166

DOI: 10.1017/9781009261159

First published 2024

A catalogue record for this publication is available from the British Library.

Library of Congress Cataloging-in-Publication Data
Names: Jadeja, Neville M., 1986- author. | Rossi, Kyle C., author.
Title: Critical care EEG basics : rapid bedside EEG reading for acute care providers /
    Neville M. Jadeja, University of Massachusetts Medical School, Massachusetts,
    Kyle C. Rossi, University of Massachusetts Medical School, Massachusetts.
Description: Cambridge, United Kingdom ; New York, NY : Cambridge University
    Press, 2023. | Includes bibliographical references and index.
Identifiers: LCCN 2023031153 (print) | LCCN 2023031154 (ebook) |
    ISBN 9781009261166 (paperback) | ISBN 9781009261159 (ebook)
Subjects: LCSH: Electroencephalography. | Critical care medicine.
Classification: LCC RC386.6.E43 J33 2023 (print) | LCC RC386.6.E43 (ebook) |
    DDC 616.8/047547–dc23/eng/20230817
LC record available at https://lccn.loc.gov/2023031153
LC ebook record available at https://lccn.loc.gov/2023031154

ISBN 978-1-009-26116-6 Paperback

NMJ dedicates this book to Shilpa Deshmukh.

KCR dedicates this book to Megan Rossi.

Contents

Foreword

The EEG, one of the oldest diagnostic tools for evaluating brain function, has now been in use for 100 years since its invention by Hans Berger. There has been a renaissance in EEG use as a means of evaluating and monitoring critically ill patients in the past 20 years, made possible by advances in computing and visualization technologies. Therefore, although EEG is a relatively ancient tool, it is simultaneously a young field. In particular, continuous EEG monitoring in the ICU has markedly improved the management of neurocritically ill patients.

There are several comprehensive textbooks, handbooks, and atlases dedicated to critical care EEG monitoring, as well as new chapters in classical EEG tomes. This can be particularly intimidating to medical professionals whose backgrounds are not in clinical neurophysiology or epilepsy, but who are nonetheless expected to utilize these tools in everyday practice. Practitioners may not even have more than a passing familiarity with EEGs themselves. This is where the new book by Neville Jadeja and Kyle Rossi becomes a valuable asset in learning critical care EEG that is both efficient and practical.

The book is short enough that it can be read cover-to-cover within a couple of days of concerted effort, even less with some familiarity with EEGs. Nonetheless, it is comprehensive enough that it should cover most of the common scenarios encountered by caretakers of the critically ill patients. The book introduces the basics of EEG recordings, when and how to order an EEG, and the importance of recognizing and accounting for recording artifacts and medication effects. The core principles of critical care EEGs – ranging from interictal epileptiform discharges to rhythmic and periodic discharges, the ictal–interictal continuum, seizures, and status epilepticus – are well covered. A special emphasis is placed on post-cardiac-arrest EEGs, which are distinct from most other critical care EEGs, and encephalopathy, which is encountered in the majority of patients undergoing critical care EEGs. As all modern EEG systems have quantitative EEG tools, this topic, too, is given special consideration, rather than detailed analysis, which can only be seen under scrutiny in retrospect.

There is a very large audience who would benefit from reading this book: the EEG technologists, nurses, advanced practice providers, non-neurology critical care physicians, and even neurocritical care physicians without specialized training in clinical neurophysiology. One of the key strengths of this book lies in its comprehensive coverage of the latest standard terminology as established by the American Clinical Neurophysiology Society. This terminology is now a cornerstone in the field, adopted by nearly all contemporary clinical neurophysiologists. Additionally, the book describes the structure of the reports generated in this discipline, enhancing the communication between the care team and the clinical neurophysiologist. This ensures a more streamlined and effective exchange of information, crucial for optimal patient care. I cannot emphasize how critical this communication is in the care of these patients, and I can think of no better way to quickly learn this language than through this very useful, readable, well-illustrated book. I warmly congratulate Drs Jadeja and Rossi on producing this outstanding work.

Jong Woo Lee, MD, PhD
Associate Professor of Neurology, Harvard Medical School
Department of Neurology, Brigham and Women's Hospital

Preface

Electroencephalograms (EEG) are commonplace in acute care environments such as emergency rooms, intensive care units, and hospital floors. Critically ill patients with altered mental status are at a high risk of seizures, which may occur without clinically apparent convulsions (nonconvulsive seizures) and therefore can only be diagnosed on EEG. Delay in the detection and treatment of continuous seizures (status epilepticus) is associated with refractoriness to therapy and secondary neurological injury. Additionally, the EEG may help confirm encephalopathy, grade its severity, characterize paroxysmal events, and titrate anesthetics and sedation, among other indications, in critically ill patients.

However, most acute care providers (including many neurologists) are unfamiliar with critical care EEG despite easy availability and widespread use. Without confident bedside EEG reading skills, they are dependent on official reports or remote interpretations, which can be difficult to understand or not immediately available for review. This pocketbook introduces the reader to the basics of critical care EEG with an emphasis on *real-time bedside EEG reading*.

Tailored specifically for acute care providers without an EEG background, this book allows readers of all skill levels to become familiar with common critical care EEG patterns and what they mean and what to do about them. With practice, quick and easy bedside EEG reading will become a powerful extension to your neurological assessment. We hope that this unique book, which is easy to understand and heavily illustrated, will help you to harness the immense potential of this fascinating test in order to best help your patients.

Acknowledgments

This approach borrows heavily from those of our teachers at the Brigham and Women's Hospital and Beth Israel Deaconess Medical Center, Harvard Medical School. We also gratefully acknowledge our colleagues at UMass Memorial Medical Center, UMass Chan Medical School, including Don Chin; Felicia Chu, MD; Ika Noviawaty, MD; Mugdha Mohanty, MD; and Brian Silver, MD. Last but not least, we thank Catherine Barnes, Kim Ingram, Beth Sexton, Ruth Swan, Marijasintha Srinivasan, and the team at Cambridge University Press for making this work possible.

How to Read This Book

This book has two parts that should be read sequentially:

Part I (Introduction) describes the basics of EEG (emphasizing critical care EEG). Additionally, it includes clinical indications for EEG, an approach to rapid bedside EEG reading, how to recognize artifact and medication effects, how to explain rhythmic or periodic patterns, and the increasingly relevant concept of the ictal-interictal continuum (IIC). It also describes how to diagnose seizures and status epilepticus as well as post–cardiac arrest patterns and quantitative EEG.

Part II (Case-Based Approach to Specific Conditions) describes an approach to specific commonly encountered ICU conditions using case-based clinical reasoning. Each case consists of a short clinical vignette that includes a brief clinical description, sample EEG, and what to do next with relevant clinical reasoning. This provides a direct practical approach to common critical care EEG patterns.

Finally, there is an appendix about understanding EEG reports. This explains the common presentation and meaning of terms used in an EEG report for acute care providers of all specialties.

Introduction

EEG Basics

1

- How EEGs are recorded
- Three rules of polarity
- Parts of an EEG machine
- Electrodes
- Montages and localization

- Display
- Frequency
- Rhythm
- Normal adult EEG
- Strengths and limitations of EEG

This chapter introduces the basic concepts of electroencephalography (EEG) recording, with which readers need to be familiar before advancing. Specifically tailored to acute care providers, it assumes that most readers do not have prior EEG reading experience. Therefore, the neurophysiology has been simplified to the "bare basics." This chapter is intended as a foundation to understand further concepts described in this book; it cannot serve as a detailed reference, for which many excellent textbooks are available.

How EEGs Are Recorded

Electroencephalographs (EEGs) are graphical representations of continuous synaptic activity of the *pyramidal neurons* in the superficial cortex. These neurons are arranged radially, like spokes of a wheel, with their superficial ends towards the cortical surface. Each neuron also functions as a dipole, with each of its two ends carrying a small but opposing charge. Summations of tiny superficial charges form cortical potentials. Electrodes placed on the scalp can measure the potential of the underlying cortical region.

When electrodes are paired, the potential difference between two electrodes (V) causes a small current (I) to move across the resistance of the circuit (R) governed by *Ohm's law* ($V = I \times R$). The strength and direction of the current are computed by the EEG machine and displayed as a waveform over time. Inputs from deeper structures, such as the thalamus, synchronize cortical neuronal activity to generate patterns of electrographic activity called rhythms.

Since synaptic transmission occurs constantly, the normal EEG is always continuous. Disruptions to neuronal function and synaptic transmission will lead to breaks in the recording (discontinuity). Therefore, discontinuity indicates cortical neuronal dysfunction.

Three Rules of Polarity

The EEG screen shows an arrangement of channels, each showing a line with waveforms. Each *channel* consists of two electrodes that record the electrical potential from their underlying region of cortex. The EEG machine then computes the potential difference between those two electrodes and displays it as a waveform.

Three simple rules of polarity govern the appearance of each waveform.

Consider, for example, a single EEG channel, say D1-D2. This is composed of scalp electrodes D1 and D2, each sampling an area of underlying cortex. Depending on their arrangement, they may lie adjacent to or distant from another. The appearance of a waveform in channel D1-D2 will depend on the relative difference in electrical potentials at electrode D1 and electrode D2 (i.e., D1 – D2). The greater the difference, the higher the amplitude (voltage). Further, the direction (polarity) of the wave is determined as follows:

- Rule 1: If potential at D1 is less than D2 (i.e., D1 < D2 or D1 is relatively negative), their difference is negative – reflecting as an upward deflection.
- Rule 2: If potential at D1 is greater than D2 (i.e., D1 > D2 or D2 is relatively negative), their difference is positive – reflecting as a downward deflection.
- Rule 3: If both D1 and D2 are equipotential or inactive, then their difference is neutral – there is no deflection.

As you can see, the pointer simply deflects to the relatively smaller (i.e., more negative, or less positive) electrode potential as shown in Figure 1.1.

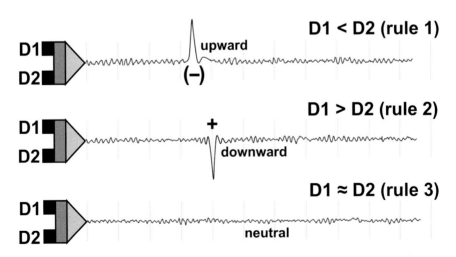

Figure 1.1 Three rules of polarity.

Parts of an EEG Machine

A typical EEG recording consists of electrodes (fixed to the patient's scalp), each of which is connected by wire to a head box. The head box is plugged into a portable computer with a display screen. It can be easily unplugged to temporarily disconnect the recording for transport.

Electrodes

These are small, circular, dome-shaped metallic discs perforated by a small hole on their top. They are applied to the scalp using glue or collodion. Collodion is extremely flammable and emits a noxious odor, but forms strong, sweat resistant, and durable connections, useful for continuous EEG.

Electrodes are made of paramagnetic materials such as stainless steel or tin and coated with silver or silver chloride. MRI conditional electrodes are also available.

Single use electrodes should be used in patients with suspected prion disease (e.g., Jakob–Creutzfeldt Disease) [1].

Application of Electrodes

First, the electrode is dipped in an adhesive paste and then placed on prepared skin. Next, a gauze soaked in collodion is placed over the electrode and air dried to form durable connections. Finally, each electrode is filled with electroconductive gel through the small hole on the top of its dome using a blunt needle and syringe. This ensures an adhesive electrical connection.

Placement of Electrodes

Electrodes are placed using the *standardized international 10–20 system*. This system uses three bony anatomical landmarks of the scalp to form a flexible map. These include the nasion (center of the nose bridge), inion (center of the occipital prominence), and preauricular point (just in front of the tragus). Points for electrode placement are selected at approximations of either 10% or 20% of the distance between the landmarks as shown below.

Each electrode is referenced by a letter representing the underlying region of cortex (e.g., frontopolar (Fp), frontal (F), temporal (T), parietal (P), occipital (O), or central (C)), and a number – even (2, 4, 6, 8) for right, odd (1, 3, 5, 7) for left, and Z for the midline (Fz, Cz, and Pz). For example, Fp1 is for the left frontopolar electrode, etc.

A common adaptation called the modified combinatorial nomenclature uses T7 for T3, T8 for T4, P7 for T5, and P8 for T6 [2]. This brings the names of these electrodes in line with the more extensive 10–10 system, which uses far more electrodes. Figures 1.2(a) and 1.2(b) show the placement of electrodes using the international 10–20 system.

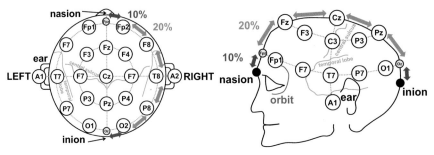

Figure 1.2(a) International 10–20 system; top view.

Figure 1.2(b) International 10–20 system; side view.

Montages and Localization

Montages

Channels (electrode pairs) are displayed on the EEG screen using specific arrangements. These specific arrangements are called *montages*.

There are many different types of montages, detailed descriptions of which are beyond the scope of this book. However, acute care providers should be familiar with using a longitudinal bipolar (double banana) montage, as this is a common default montage and easy to use at the bedside. All EEG examples in this book use this montage.

Each channel of a longitudinal bipolar montage shows the potential difference between two adjacent electrodes on the scalp, and is connected to other channels in longitudinal (front to back) chains as shown below [3].

Figure 1.3(a) shows an example of the longitudinal bipolar montage, while Figure 1.3(b) shows a schematic representation of its electrode chains.

Localization

This is the art of approximating the location (origin) of a waveform on the cortical surface.

Ideally, different types of montages should be used together during localization, but this can be challenging at the bedside. Therefore, we limit ourselves here to using the longitudinal bipolar montage.

The key to localization is an electrographic principle called a *phase reversal*. This is a simultaneous but opposite deflection in two adjacent EEG channels containing a common electrode. A phase reversal implies that the cortical potential is maximal at the location of the common electrode.

Most phase reversals are negative (><), though rarely positive phase reversals (<>) may occur. Figure 1.4 shows an example of localizing a focal sharp wave.

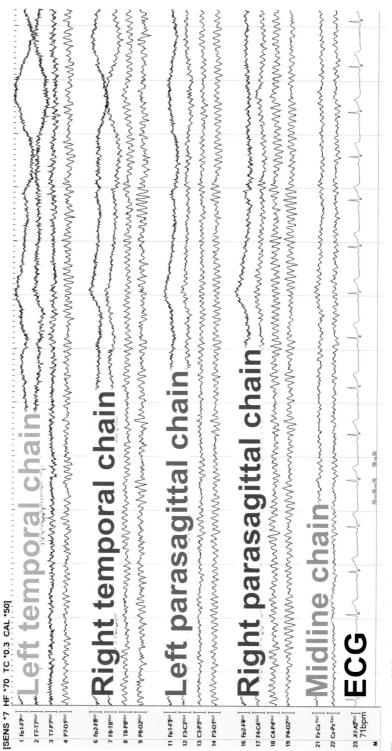

[SENS *7   HF *70 TC *0.3 CAL *50]

1 Fp1-F7(5uV)
2 F7-T7(5uV)
3 T7-P7(5uV)
4 P7-O7(5uV)

Left temporal chain

6 Fp2-F8(5uV)
7 F8-T8(5uV)
8 T8-P8(5uV)
9 P8-O2(5uV)

Right temporal chain

11 Fp1-F3(5uV)
12 F3-C3(5uV)
13 C3-P3(5uV)
14 P3-O1(5uV)

Left parasagittal chain

16 Fp2-F4(5uV)
17 F4-C4(5uV)
18 C4-P4(5uV)
19 P4-O2(5uV)

Right parasagittal chain

21 Fz-Cz(5uV)
22 Cz-Pz(5uV)

Midline chain

23 X1-X2(5uV)
71bpm

ECG

M

Figure 1.3(a) EEG in longitudinal bipolar montage.

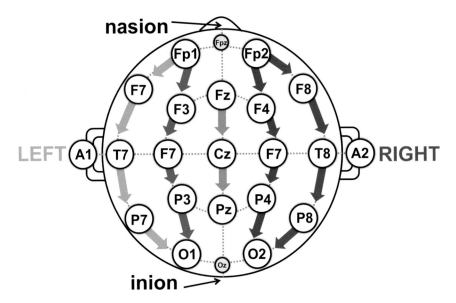

Figure 1.3(b) Longitudinal bipolar montage electrode chains.

Display (Parameters)

A typical bedside display using a longitudinal bipolar montage is shown in Figure 1.3(a). Variations to this format exist. Commonly, the left and the right temporal chains are stacked together followed by the left and right parasagittal chains. This makes it easy to compare the temporal and parasagittal regions of both hemispheres for asymmetry. Readers should know that the temporal regions are also the most epileptogenic so focusing on these channels yields results! The top bar of a recording shows the sensitivity, filter settings, and time base.

Sensitivity (μV/mm) is the magnification of EEG activity. The lower the value, the higher the amplitude of the waveform on the screen. Most EEGs are displayed at a sensitivity of 7 μV/mm as a default setting.

Frequency filters aim to reduce artifact or noise. The three common types of filters are high frequency filter (HFF), low frequency filter (LFF), and notch filter (60 Hz).

- High frequency filters (HFF) screen out frequencies greater than their setting and allow lower frequencies to pass (low pass). They are particularly useful to filter out myogenic (muscle) artifact but may alter the underlying activity to look falsely sharper. The HFF is usually set at 70 Hz.
- Low frequency filters (LFF) screen out frequencies lower than their setting and allow higher frequencies to pass (high pass).
- Notch filters are specific to screen out 60 Hz artifact.

Most displays show 10 or 15 seconds per page of EEG. Figure 1.5 shows a typical display using the longitudinal bipolar montage with excessive muscle artifact before (a) and after (b) application of 30 Hz high frequency filter.

Frequency

This refers to the number of waves occurring per second. It is measured in hertz (Hz). For example, if a rhythmic wave pattern occurs every second, its frequency is 1 Hz.

Activity can be easily described based on increasing order of frequency as follows:

- Delta range (1–4 Hz)
- Theta range (5–7 Hz)
- Alpha range (8–13 Hz)
- Beta range (>13 Hz).

Rhythm

This refers to an electrographic pattern that not only has a regular frequency, but also a specific shape and location. While frequency is merely a descriptive term, rhythms indicate normal or pathological significance – i.e., is it a normal or abnormal pattern?

For example, the "alpha rhythm" (a.k.a. posterior dominant rhythm) is an electrographic hallmark of normal wakefulness.

Normal Adult EEG

The normal background depends on the physiological state: awake, drowsy, or asleep.

Awake

Look for the *alpha rhythm (posterior dominant rhythm, PDR)*. This is the 8.5–13 Hz (alpha range) rhythm, maximal in the posterior head regions, that attenuates with eye opening (an indication of reactivity). The alpha rhythm is an obvious feature of normal wakefulness and is best observed after eye closure in the occipital channels (O). Lower amplitude *beta* activity occurs anteriorly. Any intrusion of theta or delta activity during full wakefulness is usually indicative of an abnormality. Furthermore, the amplitude of the background activity should normally decrease from posterior (O) to anterior (Fp). This is called the normal *anterior–posterior (AP) gradient*. Additionally, there will be artifact from *eye blinks* and *muscle* activity in the frontalis and temporalis muscles. Figure 1.6 shows an EEG during normal wakefulness.

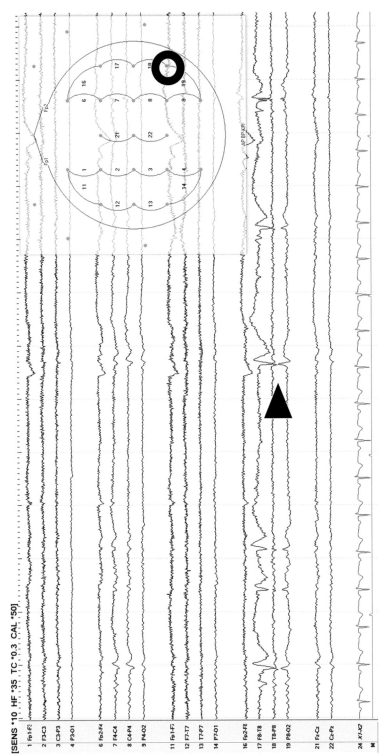

Figure 1.4 Localizing a sharp wave (black arrow) through phase reversal to electrode P8 (black circle).

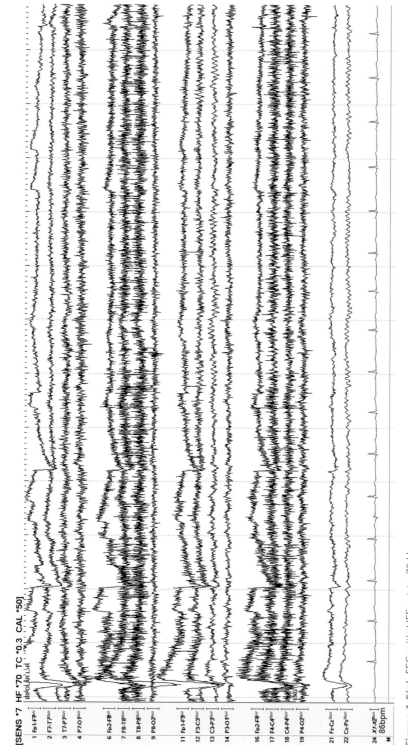

Figure 1.5(a) EEG with HFF set to 70 Hz.

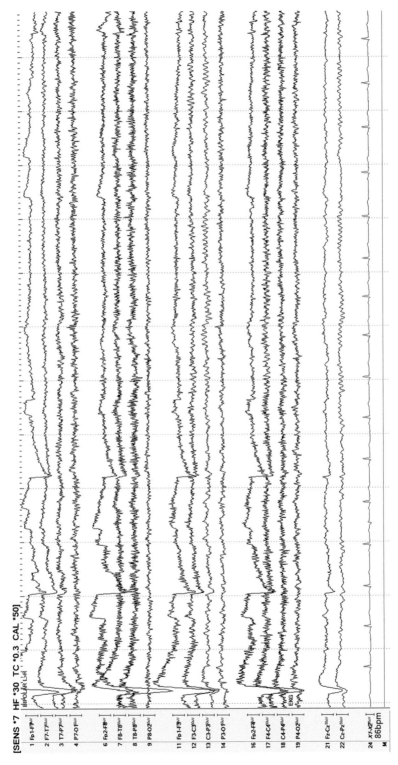

Figure 1.5(b) The same EEG with HFF set to 30 Hz.

Drowsy

As the patient becomes drowsy (N1 sleep), the *alpha rhythms can slow and become more intermittent*, the background *amplitude decreases*, the *frequency slows*, and *slow lateral ("roving") eye movements* can appear. Eye blinks and muscle artifact disappear. Figure 1.7 shows the EEG during drowsiness.

Sleep

Light sleep shows further slowing of the background frequencies. *Stage N2 sleep* is identified by the presence of **sleep spindles** and **K-complexes**. Sleep spindles are transient, frontocentral predominant, spindle-shaped bursts of 12–16 Hz activity, while K-complexes are composed of a high amplitude, centrally predominant, generalized wave, often followed by a brief burst of spindle activity. Figure 1.8(a) shows stage N2 sleep.

Stage N3 or *slow wave sleep* is characterized by high amplitude, generalized, semirhythmic delta slowing [4]. Rapid eye movement (REM) sleep is seldom seen in the ICU. Figure 1.8(b) shows stage N3 or slow wave sleep.

Strengths and Limitations of EEG

Strengths

The EEG is a noninvasive and easily available test to evaluate cortical function. Further, it has excellent temporal (time) resolution. This means that though it is not nearly as good as neuroimaging in pointing to the location of problems (low spatial resolution), it can almost immediately (in milliseconds) detect any alteration of cortical function.

Additionally, EEG accompanied by video recording remains the gold standard test for the diagnosis of seizures.

Limitations

Relatively low spatial resolution aside, EEG has other limitations. It has poor resolution for neuronal activities that arise from deeper structures of the brain such as the sulcal depths, the insulae, as well as basal and mesial structures. Remember, the cortex is deeply enfolded and most of it does not lie on the surface!

Further, cortical potentials measured at the scalp are tiny (often only a few microvolts) due to the dampening effect of thick skull bones, fluid, and fascia. Therefore, a sizeable region of cortex must be involved to produce scalp signals (by some estimates, around 6–10 cm^2). For this reason, smaller

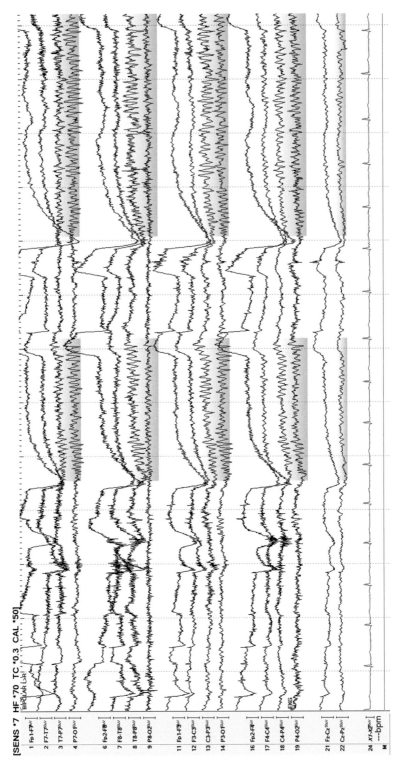

Figure 1.6 Normal awake EEG; the PDR is highlighted in red.

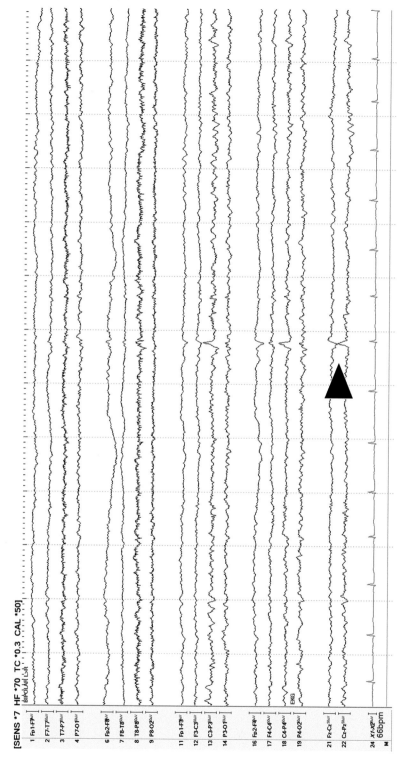

Figure 1.7 Normal drowsy EEG; black arrow marks a normal "vertex wave."

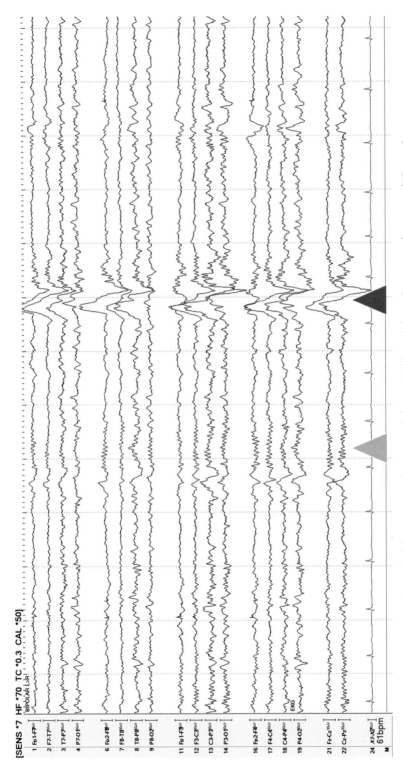

Figure 1.8(a) Normal stage N2 sleep; the blue arrow marks a normal sleep spindle, and the red arrow marks a normal K-complex.

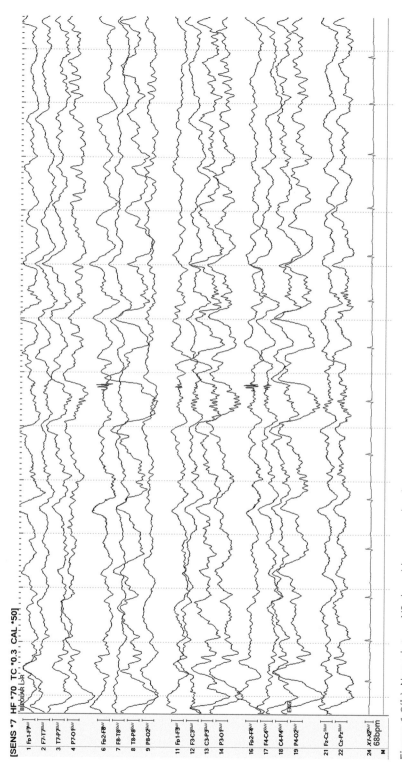

Figure 1.8(b) Normal stage N3 sleep (slow wave sleep).

foci of activity, such as seizure onsets, may not always be detected on scalp recordings. However, they may still lead to clinical manifestations such as epileptic aura or focal motor seizures. Generally, *if awareness is impaired (e.g., unresponsiveness during a seizure), then the EEG is abnormal.* This is likely because a large region of cortical dysfunction is required for an impairment of awareness.

References

1. Eggenberger E. Prion disease. *Neurologic Clinics.* 2007 Aug 1;25(3):833–42.
2. Acharya JN, Hani AJ, Cheek J, Thirumala P, Tsuchida TN. American Clinical Neurophysiology Society Guideline 2: Guidelines for Standard Electrode Position Nomenclature. *The Neurodiagnostic Journal.* 2016 Oct 1;56(4):245–52.
3. Acharya JN, Hani AJ, Thirumala P, Tsuchida TN. American Clinical Neurophysiology Society Guideline 3: A Proposal for Standard Montages to Be Used in Clinical EEG. *The Neurodiagnostic Journal.* 2016 Oct 1;56(4):253–60.
4. Tatum IV WO, Husain AM, Benbadis SR, Kaplan PW. Normal adult EEG and patterns of uncertain significance. *Journal of Clinical Neurophysiology.* 2006 Jun 1;23(3):194–207.

Introduction

Indications

2

- When to request an EEG
- Limitations of critical care EEG
- Continuous vs. routine EEG
- Duration of monitoring
- Advantages of bedside EEG reading

The most important indication for EEG in critically ill patients is to evaluate fluctuating or persistently abnormal mental status (or other focal neurological deficits) that cannot otherwise be explained. Commonly, these symptoms are a manifestation of physiological diffuse cerebral dysfunction (encephalopathy), or they may be due to seizure activity without apparent clinical manifestations. Such "nonconvulsive" seizures (NCS), that may only be detected by EEG, occur in at least 8–10% of critically ill patients [1]. Continuous or frequent NCS are called nonconvulsive status epilepticus (NCSE) and may result in secondary neurological injury, including neuronal death or alteration of neuronal networks [2]. Left untreated, NCSE can become refractory to treatment [3]. Further, delays in diagnosis and longer duration of NCSE are associated with poor outcomes, increased mortality, and chronic sequelae such as cognitive impairment and epilepsy [4,5]. Therefore, timely EEG is essential for early detection and treatment [6].

When to Request an EEG
- Acute brain injuries
- Altered mental status (without acute brain injury)
- After convulsive status epilepticus (CSE)
- Generalized tonic clonic seizures (GTC), without return to baseline
- Management of refractory status epilepticus
- Monitoring depth of anesthesia/sedation
- Paroxysmal clinical events concerning for seizure
- Pharmacological paralysis
- Post cardiac arrest
- Brain death evaluation

Acute Brain Injuries (e.g., Trauma, Hemorrhage, Ischemia, and Encephalitis)

NCS/SE is common after acute brain injuries. Severe injuries result in greater seizure risk. Empiric antiseizure drug prophylaxis may not be adequate for seizure prevention. Additionally, EEG monitoring may be useful to detect delayed cerebral ischemia (DCI) and aid in prognostication [6,7].

Altered Mental Status (without Acute Brain Injury)

NCS/SE is a risk in critically ill patients with altered mentation, even if there is no prior history of brain injury or epilepsy. The elderly and those with severe sepsis, hepatic encephalopathy, and uremic encephalopathy are especially vulnerable. Additionally, EEG can confirm encephalopathy, grade its severity, suggest potential etiologies, and estimate prognosis. Unexpectedly normal EEG in coma may suggest locked-in syndrome, catatonia, or psychogenic coma [6,7].

After Convulsive Status Epilepticus (CSE) or Generalized Tonic Clonic (GTC) Seizures without Return to Baseline

Continuous or frequent convulsions without recovery are termed CSE. CSE is a clinical diagnosis that does not require EEG. In fact, the record is obscured by muscle artifact. However, EEG is crucial in those who do not recover immediately after cessation of motor activity. This is because NCS/SE is common after CSE with one study reporting NCS in 48% and NCSE in 14% in the first 24 hours after CSE [8]. Additionally, EEG is useful to distinguish NCS/SE from prolonged postictal encephalopathy or sedative effect. An unexpectedly normal record during convulsions may suggest functional/psychogenic SE [6,7].

Management of Refractory Status Epilepticus (RSE)

RSE is the term for persistent seizures despite first line therapy with a benzodiazepine and at least one acceptable antiseizure medication (ASM); seizures occurring or recurring despite anesthesia/sedation is super-refractory SE (SRSE). Since seizure activity in these conditions is usually nonconvulsive, the EEG is necessary for management. This includes monitoring responses to antiseizure therapies, titration of anesthesia/sedation, trending rhythmic and periodic patterns, confirming seizure termination, and detecting recurrence [6,7].

Monitoring Depth of Anesthesia/Sedation

The EEG can augment a bedside assessment of consciousness during anesthesia/sedation. It can determine adequacy of burst suppression (a depth of sedation often necessary for RSE) or complete suppression in medically induced coma (e.g., pentobarbital coma) [6,7].

Paroxysmal Clinical Events Concerning for Seizure

Paroxysms such as abnormal movements (e.g., eyelid flutter, nystagmus, chewing, myoclonus, twitches, tremors, rigors, and posturing), dysautonomia spells (e.g., apnea, heart rate, and blood pressure changes), or unexplained elevations in intracranial pressure are common in critically ill patients. EEG is useful for detecting if these are due to seizure [6].

Pharmacological Paralysis

The EEG is useful for detecting seizures during periods of neuromuscular blockade (e.g., during extracorporeal membrane oxygenation (ECMO) or therapeutic hypothermia (TH)), as motor activity is suppressed [6].

Post Cardiac Arrest (CA)

Seizures (usually nonconvulsive) occur in a third of comatose patients after cardiac arrest. EEG is recommended during periods of TH and rewarming. Additionally, EEG can distinguish cortical from subcortical myoclonus and aid in neurological prognostication [6,7].

Brain Death (Death by Neurological Criteria)

The EEG may be used as a supplementary tool to confirm a diagnosis of brain death. Importantly, the EEG should not be used alone to determine brain death [9].

Limitations of Critical Care EEG

Compared to the controlled environment of a neurophysiology laboratory, recording EEGs in critical care settings (e.g., ICUs, emergency rooms, step down units, and hospital floors) presents challenges:

1. **Artifact** can often arise due to contamination from electrical noise coming from various devices in the patient's room (e.g., IV pumps, dialysis machines, and even the bed!). Critical care settings are also busy places with frequent movement of equipment, patients, and staff, making the record prone to various other artifacts.
2. **Electrode placement** is hampered by scalp lesions (e.g., hematomas, infections, or swellings) and surgical wounds and dressings (e.g., craniotomy). Electrodes become contaminated by blood or discharge. Even sweaty skin causes artifact.
3. **Patient movements** (e.g., during personal care, transfers, or volitional) can disrupt recordings and introduce artifact. The critically ill are prone to many abnormal movements or paroxysms that can mimic seizures. Agitated or delirious patients may pull off their electrodes or self-disconnect the recording entirely.

4. **Portable EEG machines** may be (mis)handled, with cables accidentally disconnected during transfers. The video camera may be inadvertently focused away from the patient.
5. **Prolonged recording** lasting several days can result in loss of electrode integrity and cause skin erosions. In severe cases, scalp blisters or pressure ulcers may form.

Critical care EEG can add enormous clinical value despite all these limitations. With sufficient practice, readers will become comfortable recognizing various artifacts and making accurate bedside interpretations [6,7,10].

Continuous vs. Routine EEG

Two types of EEG are commonly used in critical care settings – continuous and routine. Readers should use the same approach to bedside interpretation for both types. Both may be accompanied by video for clinical correlation. They differ in their duration and application of electrodes. Acute care providers should know which test to request for their patient depending on the pros and cons of each type.

Continuous EEG (CEEG) refers to prolonged recordings (many hours to days) in hospitalized patients. Graphical displays of quantitative EEG (QEEG) trends may be included. Often, CEEG electrodes are affixed with collodion. Alternatively, a tight head wrap can be used. CEEG is often referred to as "long-term monitoring" (LTM).

Routine EEG (REEG) is typically only about 20–60 minutes per study. REEG electrodes are usually affixed with glue or tape. Serial REEGs can also be performed if CEEG is not available or is not tolerated by the patient. Routine EEG may also be referred to as a "portable EEG", when performed using a portable machine.

Making the Correct Choice

Continuous EEG is preferred for most indications in critically ill patients. This is because continuous recordings of at least 24–48 hours will identify about 80–95% of those with NCS. In comparison, REEGs identify NCS in only 45–58% of those in whom seizures would be eventually recorded [11].

Additionally, CEEG allows optimal monitoring of the evolution (progressive change) of rhythmic and periodic patterns (RPPs), seizure semiology, therapeutic response to antiseizure medications (ASMs), titration of anesthesia/sedation, and capture and characterization of paroxysmal events. Continuous EEG with quantitative analysis (QEEG) is useful to detect delayed cerebral ischemia (DCI) in comatose patients after subarachnoid hemorrhage (SAH). However, CEEG is costly, labor intensive, and not easily available outside of specialized centers.

Routine EEGs are better tolerated (especially in delirious or agitated patients), easily available, and less resource intensive. As REEGs are shorter, artifact generating activities such as suctioning or repositioning may also be temporarily avoided to improve the study quality. They are useful for short baseline or follow-up assessment.

If CEEG is indicated but unavailable, transfer to a specialized center should be considered in the appropriate circumstances [6,7].

Duration of Monitoring

For most indications, at least 24 hours of CEEG recording is sufficient to exclude NCS/SE. However, the duration of CEEG monitoring should be individually tailored to the patient based on prior seizure history, clinical exam, initial EEG findings, and overall clinical course:

1. Duration of CEEG should be extended (48–72 hours) in those with prior seizures, coma, pharmacological sedation, and initial high risk findings on EEG such as periodic discharges (GPDs, LPDs), lateralized rhythmic delta activity (LRDA), and brief potentially ictal rhythmic discharges (BIRDs), as NCS/SE may be delayed [12].
2. For non-comatose patients without prior seizures, about 30–60 minutes of recording (REEG) with no epileptogenic (high risk) EEG patterns sufficiently predicts a less than 5% risk of seizures in the following 72 hours. However, if high risk EEG patterns are detected, the study should be extended (48–72 hours) [13].
3. Recordings should generally be continued for at least 24 hours after seizure control is achieved, as risk of recurrence is greatest during that time. Also, continue recording during intravenous administration of antiseizure medications and for (at least) another 24 hours after these are stopped (longer if medications have very long half-lives).
4. Recommendations for CEEG in comatose patients after SAH include starting before the highest risk of vasospasm (typically day 3 post SAH) and continuing until this risk has subsided (day 14 post SAH). For post–cardiac arrest coma, CEEG should begin during TH and continue after rewarming [6,7].

Advantages of Bedside EEG Reading

The digital display screen of an EEG machine can be easily viewed (and read) while recording at the bedside. Though only a brief snapshot of the entire recording, bedside reading provides a valuable opportunity to interpret brain function and recognize important EEG patterns in real time.

Additionally, the reader may opt to pause the recording and review it entirely or in selected parts for a more detailed assessment.

We will refer to these practices as bedside EEG reading.

Advantages – Why Read This Book?

1. Bedside EEG is a powerful extension of the neurological examination. Almost instantly, the reader has objective and actionable information to

guide their clinical reasoning such as confirmation of encephalopathy, diagnosis, and management of NCS/SE. Additionally, QEEG (if available) is useful to trend patterns over time.

2. A wealth of supplementary information such as potential etiology, severity, and prognostication can be gained by a skillful reader. Serial comparisons allow monitoring for neurological improvement/deterioration.

3. EEG reactivity (EEG-R) can be tested at the bedside and provides additional prognostic value (see Chapter 3).

4. Together with the neurological exam, bedside reading serves as a point of care tool to estimate depth of anesthesia/sedation.

5. Acute care providers (who are skillful readers) become less dependent on remote interpretations that may not always be immediately available, even at specialized centers.

6. Furthermore, bedside reading by acute care providers also complements reporting by qualified electroencephalographers for the following reasons:
   - Sources of artifact that contaminate critical care recordings are easier to identify at bedside.
   - Conversely, abnormal physiology (e.g., nystagmus) or even seizures that may be misdiagnosed as "artifact" can be reevaluated at the bedside.
   - Concurrent video recordings may be unreliable in certain situations such as when clinical behaviors are subtle, clinical interactions that help assess the patient's mental status are not performed, or the camera is focused away from the patient or absent.

Therefore, bedside EEG reading is a useful skill for acute care providers. Skillful readers can reduce diagnostic delays, implement timely management, and potentially improve patient outcomes [14,15].

Limitations

Acute care providers should not use bedside reading to replace reporting by qualified electroencephalographers. Interpretations based on a brief look at the recording **do not** substitute for a detailed review of an entire recording (especially for CEEG). When in doubt, acute care providers should always seek clarification from an experienced electroencephalographer, especially when making clinical decisions.

However, knowing when to call for help (a benefit of bedside reading) can be as important as making that call!

References

1. Towne AR, Waterhouse EJ, Boggs JG, et al. Prevalence of nonconvulsive status epilepticus in comatose patients. *Neurology.* 2000 Jan 25;54(2):340.
2. Trinka E, Cock H, Hesdorffer D, et al. A definition and classification of status epilepticus – Report of the ILAE Task Force on Classification of Status Epilepticus. *Epilepsia.* 2015 Oct;56(10):1515–23.

3. Betjemann JP, Lowenstein DH. Status epilepticus in adults. *The Lancet Neurology.* 2015 Jun 1;14(6):615–24.
4. Young BG, Jordan KG, Doig GS. An assessment of nonconvulsive seizures in the intensive care unit using continuous EEG monitoring: An investigation of variables associated with mortality. *Neurology.* 1996 Jul 1;47(1):83–9.
5. Punia V, Bena J, Krishnan B, Newey C, Hantus S. New onset epilepsy among patients with periodic discharges on continuous electroencephalographic monitoring. *Epilepsia.* 2018 Aug;59(8):1612–20.
6. Herman ST, Abend NS, Bleck TP, et al. Consensus statement on continuous EEG in critically ill adults and children, Part I: Indications. *Journal of Clinical Neurophysiology.* 2015 Apr;32(2):87.
7. Claassen J, Taccone FS, Horn P, Holtkamp M, Stocchetti N, Oddo M. Recommendations on the use of EEG monitoring in critically ill patients: Consensus statement from the neurointensive care section of the ESICM. *Intensive Care Medicine.* 2013 Aug;39(8):1337–51.
8. DeLorenzo RJ, Waterhouse EJ, Towne AR, et al. Persistent nonconvulsive status epilepticus after the control of convulsive status epilepticus. *Epilepsia.* 1998 Aug;39(8):833–40.
9. American Clinical Neurophysiology Society. Guideline 3: Minimum Technical Standards for EEG Recording in Suspected Cerebral Death. *Journal of Clinical Neurophysiology.* 2006 Apr;23(2):97–104.
10. White DM, Van Cott CA. EEG artifacts in the intensive care unit setting. *American Journal of Electroneurodiagnostic Technology.* 2010 Mar 1;50(1):8–25.
11. Claassen J, Mayer SA, Kowalski RG, Emerson RG, Hirsch LJ. Detection of electrographic seizures with continuous EEG monitoring in critically ill patients. *Neurology.* 2004 May 25;62(10):1743–8.
12. Gaspard N, Manganas L, Rampal N, Petroff OA, Hirsch LJ. Similarity of lateralized rhythmic delta activity to periodic lateralized epileptiform discharges in critically ill patients. *JAMA Neurology.* 2013 Oct 1;70(10):1288–95.
13. Crepeau AZ, Fugate JE, Mandrekar J, et al. Value analysis of continuous EEG in patients during therapeutic hypothermia after cardiac arrest. *Resuscitation.* 2014 Jun 1;85(6):785–9.
14. Lybeck A, Cronberg T, Borgquist O, et al. Bedside interpretation of simplified continuous EEG after cardiac arrest. *Acta Anaesthesiologica Scandinavica.* 2020 Jan;64(1):85–92.
15. Legriel S, Jacq G, Lalloz A, et al. Teaching important basic EEG patterns of bedside electroencephalography to critical care staffs: A prospective multicenter study. *Neurocritical Care.* 2021 Feb;34:144–53.

Chapter 3

Real-Time Bedside EEG Reading

- What to know before you begin reading
- Three easy steps for bedside EEG reading
- How to analyze the background

- Abnormal waves
- How to check for EEG reactivity
- Qualitative grading of encephalopathy

When evaluating a patient on CEEG, take a few moments to observe the record, then ask yourself two basic questions.

- **Is the patient encephalopathic?**
- **If so, is it due to epileptic activity (seizures)?**

This book enables you to answer these two fundamental questions, and then *correlate* the EEG findings with the clinical history to see if it makes sense. Of course, brief bedside reading cannot replace the report of an experienced electroencephalographer. Always look at their report and, if in doubt, seek their help!

What to Know Before You Begin Reading

Bedside analysis should be used in conjunction with a patient's history, neurological exam, laboratory results, and neuroimaging. Additionally, know what medications they are on and if they have a skull defect.

Sedatives contribute to encephalopathy; some medications may even trigger seizures.

Skull defects (e.g., craniotomy or fracture) result in loss of normal signal dampening. Therefore, EEG activity over skull defects may appear taller, faster, and sharper compared to the surrounding region (breach effect). *Avoid over-interpreting sharp waves in a skull breach region.*

Now you are ready to read the EEG!

Three Easy Steps for Bedside EEG Reading

Begin by checking the *recording parameters* (the top bar). These include montage, sensitivity, recording (paper) speed, and filters. You are familiar with these from Chapter 1, EEG Basics. Recording parameters are usually kept the same for every study while recording, but are still worth checking as minor changes may alter the appearance of the recording and confuse the reader.

Most EEGs will be displayed in a *longitudinal bipolar montage* at a sensitivity of 7–10 μV. Remember, each vertical line denotes 1 second of recording time; about 10–15 seconds of recording is displayed at a time depending on screen size.

Now, appreciate the background activity and any prominent or recurring waveforms that stand out from the surrounding activity. Usually, these "eye catching" waveforms are either artifact or abnormal waves. Let's go through this process again with three simple steps:

- **Step 1: Analyze the background.**
- **Step 2: Search for abnormal waves, if any.**
- **Step 3: (Recognize) Artifacts.**

Using this simple approach, you can quickly analyze the EEG at the bedside.

Step 1: Analyze the Background

The background refers to the baseline electrographic brain activity. It indicates the functional state of the underlying cerebral cortex. Analyzing the background can confirm encephalopathy and help grade its severity.

Evaluate the background for continuity, symmetry, voltage (amplitude), and predominant frequency. *Ask: Is there a posterior dominant rhythm (PDR)?*

Step 2: Search for Abnormal Waveforms, If Any

Abnormal waveforms stand out from the surrounding background. They may be *slow* or *sharp* waves depending on their shape. Slow waves typically suggest nonspecific focal cerebral dysfunction while sharp waves are a marker for increased seizure risk. *Do you see any slow or sharp waves? If so, are they sporadic or repetitive/rhythmic (occurring at a regular interval)?*

Step 3: Recognize Artifacts

Artifact waves are not produced by the brain. These extracerebral waves occur due to external sources (e.g., ventilator) or other body organs (e.g., eyes, muscles, heart). Recognizing artifact avoids mistaking them for abnormal cortical activity, including seizures. *Ask: Do you recognize any common artifacts?*

The remainder of this chapter provides additional guidance on analyzing the background and abnormal waveforms (Steps 1 and 2), while Chapter 4 focuses on recognizing artifacts (Step 3).

How to Analyze the Background

Background analysis is the first step to successful bedside EEG reading. Remember, analyzing the background can provide objective evidence of encephalopathy and grade its severity. Additionally, asymmetry of the background may indicate focal dysfunction (e.g., stroke, tumor, or postictal dysfunction).

Describe the background based on continuity, symmetry, voltage, predominant frequency, and presence of a PDR.

What Is Continuity?

Assess whether the recording is continuous (i.e., there are no periods of flattening (suppression) of the baseline EEG activity). A normal EEG background is always continuous.

A *discontinuous* record is one in which the baseline activity is interrupted by periods of suppression. Discontinuity is one of many electrographic hallmarks of encephalopathy. With further deterioration of consciousness and increasing discontinuity, the EEG becomes *burst suppressed* (more than half of the entire recording is flat), followed by *complete suppression*.

While occasional discontinuity may not be seen during brief analysis, burst suppression or complete suppression is easily identified at the bedside. Figure 3.1 shows burst suppression, while Figure 3.2 shows complete background suppression.

What Is Symmetry?

Compare and contrast the activity of both hemispheres. This is easy with the recording in longitudinal bipolar montage, because the left side (odd numbered) "chains" (temporal and parasagittal) usually alternate with the right side (even numbered) chains. Recall that a chain is a group of channels moving from the front to the back of the head. This allows for side-by-side comparison of left and right temporal and parasagittal chains respectively.

Specifically, check for symmetry in *voltage* (estimated height or amplitude) and *frequencies*.

Normally, both hemispheres will be similar in voltage and distribution of frequencies. Easily distinguishable *asymmetry* is usually abnormal.

Asymmetric recordings can mean either of two things:

- Decrease in voltage and/or slowing of frequency (depression) (e.g., large stroke or subdural hematoma); *or*
- Increase in voltage and/or faster frequencies (enhancement) (e.g., breach effect of craniotomy, or sometimes with seizure activity).

Therefore, asymmetric recordings can indicate the presence of either depressed activity (e.g., a structural or physiologic dysfunction) or enhanced activity (e.g., breach effect from a craniotomy) of a hemisphere.

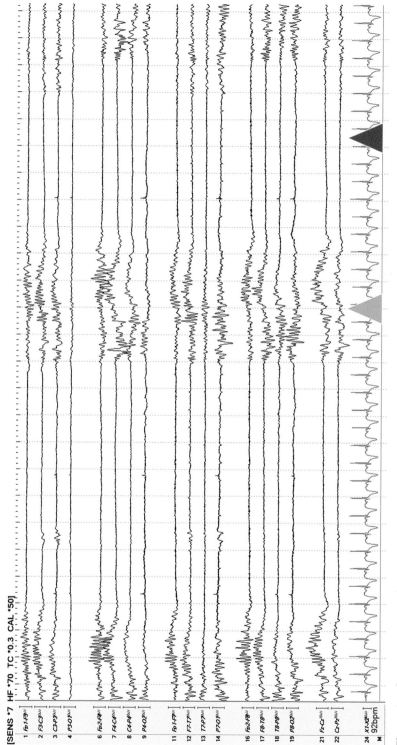

Figure 3.1 Burst suppression. The blue arrow marks a "burst," and the red arrow marks an interburst suppression. Note the compressed time scale.

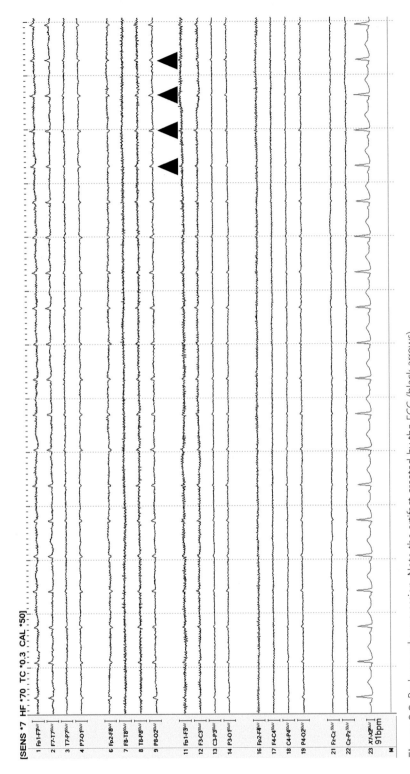

Figure 3.2 Background suppression. Note the artifact created by the ECG (black arrows).

Sometimes, a focal lesion may coexist on the side of the breach effect (e.g., craniotomy for tumor) resulting in both increased slow frequencies *and* higher voltage, faster, and sharper activity over the same hemisphere. Though difficult to perform at the bedside, a careful comparison of the hemispheric backgrounds can identify this. Figure 3.3 shows background asymmetry.

What Is Voltage?

Estimate the background voltage based on the height of the activity from peak to trough as shown in Figure 3.4. If the background is burst suppressed (discontinuous), estimate voltage of activity within bursts.

Usually, a normal voltage is greater than 20 μV. Suppression refers to periods where most activity is less than 10 μV, and attenuation refers to periods where most activity is between 10 and 20 μV. Often, persistently decreased voltage (attenuation) is suggestive of encephalopathy. The lower the voltage, the greater the severity of encephalopathy. Figure 3.4 shows a low voltage (attenuated) background.

What Is the Predominant Frequency?

Count the typical background frequency (approximate number of waves per second between the vertical lines). Normal background frequency during wakefulness is usually *alpha* (8–13 Hz). Slowing of the background frequency to *theta* (4–8 Hz) or *delta* (<4 Hz) during wakefulness is usually abnormal (encephalopathy). The degree of slowing may correlate with the severity of encephalopathy. The background normally slows during periods of drowsiness and sleep. Additionally, look for a *posterior dominant rhythm (PDR)*. Normally, the PDR is a posterior predominant *alpha rhythm* (8.5–13 Hz) that characteristically diminishes with eye opening (reactive). Slowing of the PDR followed by absence of PDR are features of mild encephalopathy [1]. Figure 3.5 shows a slow PDR indicating mild encephalopathy, while Figure 3.6 shows loss of the PDR.

Abnormal Waves

Abnormal waves are easy to identify as they stand out from the surrounding background, often disrupting it. They are described based on their *morphology (shape), location,* and *occurrence*.

Morphology

Abnormal waves can appear *blunted* (slow waves) or *pointed* (sharp waves, sharps). The most pointed sharp waves are spikes. If multiple spikes (or sharps) occur together in a cluster, they are called *polyspikes*. Spikes or sharp waves are often immediately followed by a *slow wave*; hence the complex is often called a *spike-wave* or *sharp-slow wave* discharge. Typically, spikes or sharps are associated with risk for epileptic seizures (epileptiform discharges), while slow waves suggest underlying focal cerebral dysfunction.

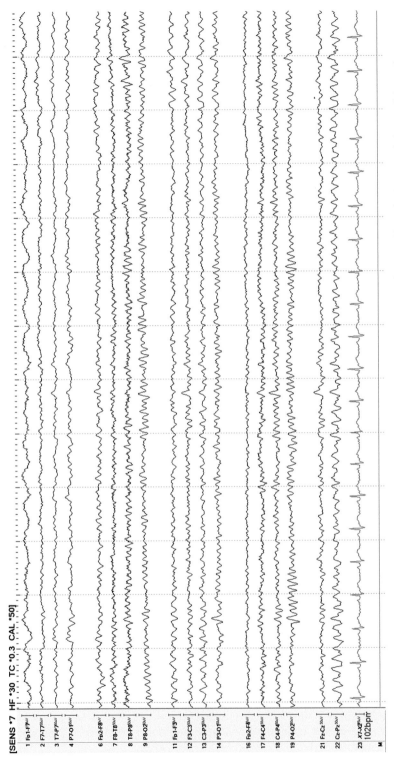

Figure 3.3 Background asymmetry: focal slowing in the left hemisphere, maximal in the temporal region. Note the increased slow activity and decreased fast activity in the left hemisphere.

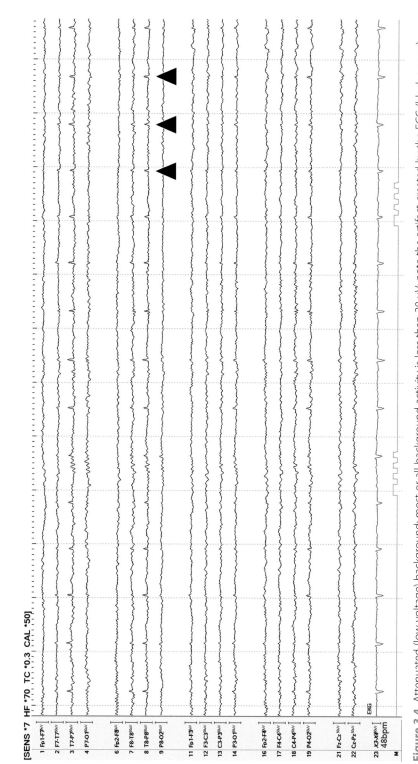

Figure 3.4 Attenuated (low voltage) background; most or all background activity is less than 20 μV; note the artifact created by the ECG (black arrows).

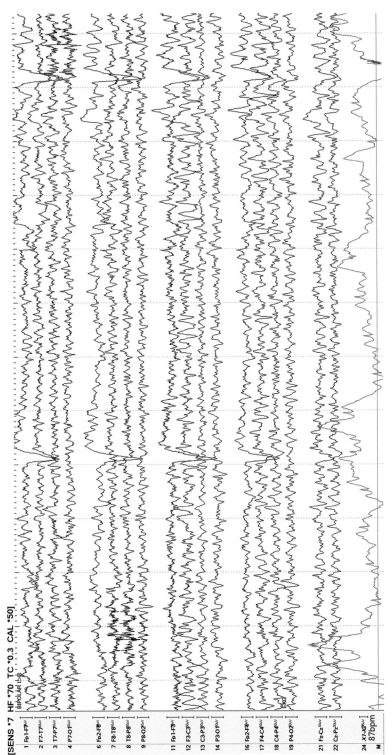

Figure 3.5 Slowing of the PDR to 6.5–7 Hz. There is also disruption of the typical anterior–posterior (AP) gradient.

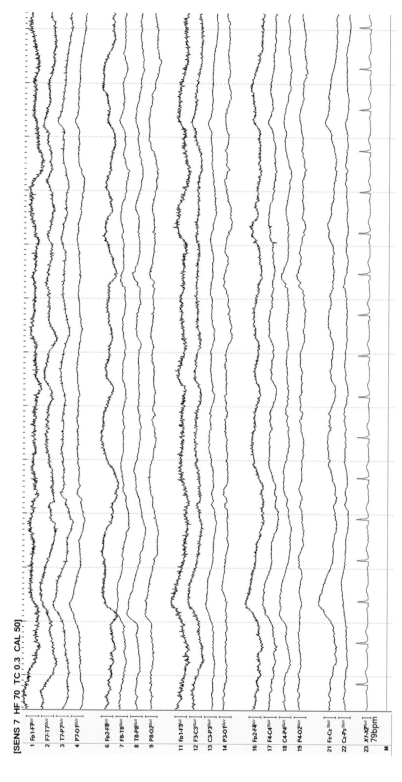

[SENS 7 HF 70 TC 0.3 CAL 50]

1 Fp1-F7⁽ᴬᵛ⁾
2 F7-T7⁽ᴮᴬᵛ⁾
3 T7-P7⁽ᴮᴬᵛ⁾
4 P7-O1⁽ᴮᴬᵛ⁾

6 Fp2-F8⁽ᴬᵛ⁾
7 F8-T8⁽ᴮᴬᵛ⁾
8 T8-P8⁽ᴮᴬᵛ⁾
9 P8-O2⁽ᴮᴬᵛ⁾

11 Fp1-F3⁽ᴬᵛ⁾
12 F3-C3⁽ᴮᴬᵛ⁾
13 C3-P3⁽ᴮᴬᵛ⁾
14 P3-O1⁽ᴮᴬᵛ⁾

16 Fp2-F4⁽ᴬᵛ⁾
17 F4-C4⁽ᴮᴬᵛ⁾
18 C4-P4⁽ᴮᴬᵛ⁾
19 P4-O2⁽ᴮᴬᵛ⁾

21 Fz-Cz⁽ᴮᴬᵛ⁾
22 Cz-Pz⁽ᴮᴬᵛ⁾

23 X1-X2⁽ᴮᴬᵛ⁾
79bpm

M

Figure 3.6 Loss of the PDR.

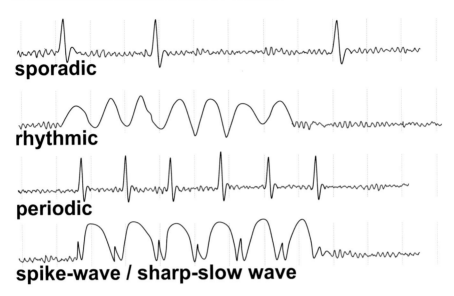

sporadic

rhythmic

periodic

spike-wave / sharp-slow wave

Figure 3.7 Patterns of abnormal waveforms.

Location

Abnormal waves may appear symmetrically over both hemispheres (*generalized*) or predominate within a single hemisphere (*lateralized*).

Occurrence

Abnormal waves occur in a *sporadic* (isolated) or *repetitive* fashion. Repetitive waveforms often have a relatively uniform appearance. They are *periodic* if they recur at nearly regular intervals between consecutive waves, or *rhythmic* if they recur at a regular interval without background between consecutive waves. Since periodic waveforms are usually sharp waves, they are termed *periodic discharges (PD)*, whereas rhythmic waveforms are usually delta waves and are termed *rhythmic delta activity (RDA)*.

This simplified description is based on the American Clinical Neurophysiology Society's standardized critical care EEG terminology [1]. Figure 3.7 shows common abnormal waveform patterns.

How to Check for Reactivity

Reactivity is a visible and reproducible *change in the background* occurring within a few seconds after *patient stimulation*. Testing for EEG reactivity (EEG-R) is a valuable benefit of bedside EEG reading in comatose patients.

Test EEG-R after reviewing the baseline record. The following standardized method to testing is recommended:

1. Apply *graded stimuli* to the undisturbed patient. Begin with an *auditory* stimulus such as clapping or calling their name followed by a *noxious* stimulus such as peripheral nail bed pressure. Additionally, visual stimuli such as passive eye opening or photic stimulation, or central pain such as sternal rub or trapezius squeeze may be used.
2. Unless reactivity is elicited, each stimulus should be applied for about 5 seconds and repeated at least three times.
3. Once reactivity is elicited, the same stimulus should be reapplied at least once for confirmation.
4. Stimulus-induced artifacts (e.g., muscle, eye blinks or spinal movements), or the emergence of rhythmic, periodic discharges and/or electrographic seizures do not qualify as reactive. To qualify as reactive, there should be a *change in the background.*

Annotate precisely the start and stopping of stimulation. Additionally, consider the degree of sedation, analgesia, and prevalent neuromuscular blockade [2]. Figure 3.8 shows a reactive background before, and Figure 3.9 after stimulation.

Clinical Significance of EEG-R
Loss of EEG-R is *diagnostic* of severe encephalopathy. Additionally, it serves as one of many *prognostic* markers in coma including after cardiac arrest.

Noxious stimuli are more effective at eliciting EEG-R compared to auditory stimuli, however both modalities should be applied as they use distinct but complementary neural pathways.

Auditory stimuli test functional integrity of the auditory pathways, while noxious (sensory) stimuli assess pain projection pathways. Visual stimuli (least effective) assess the visual pathway from the retina to the visual cortex. Overall, EEG-R assesses the function of cortical and subcortical structures of the brainstem–thalamic and cortical–thalamic loops.

Daily or serial testing is recommended, as an optimal time to perform EEG-R testing (e.g., after cardiac arrest) has not been established. Independent of etiology, those patients with normal EEG-R likely have favorable outcomes compared to those with non-reactive EEGs.

Absent EEG-R is a sensitive and specific predictor of poor neurologic outcomes when used in conjunction with other EEG patterns as part of a multimodal approach for prognostication in comatose patients after cardiac arrest. However, the presence of EEG-R alone may not reliably predict good outcomes after cardiac arrest [3–5].

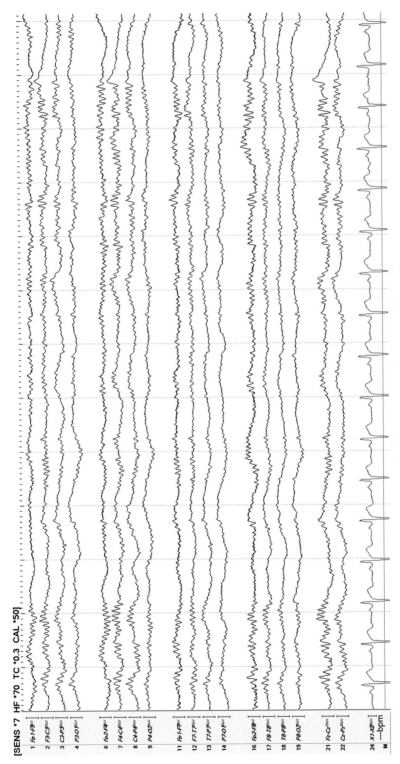

Figure 3.8 Encephalopathic (slow) background with overriding faster activity, prior to reactivity testing.

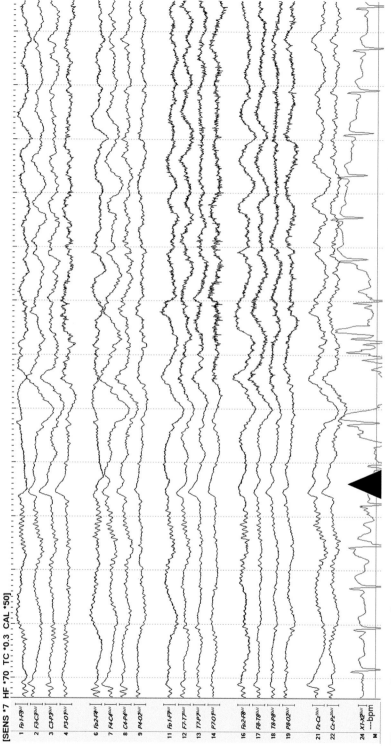

Figure 3.9 Same patient after reactivity testing (loud sound, black arrow), showing a reduction in the amount of fast activity and an increase in higher voltage slow rhythmic activity with superimposed muscle artifact.

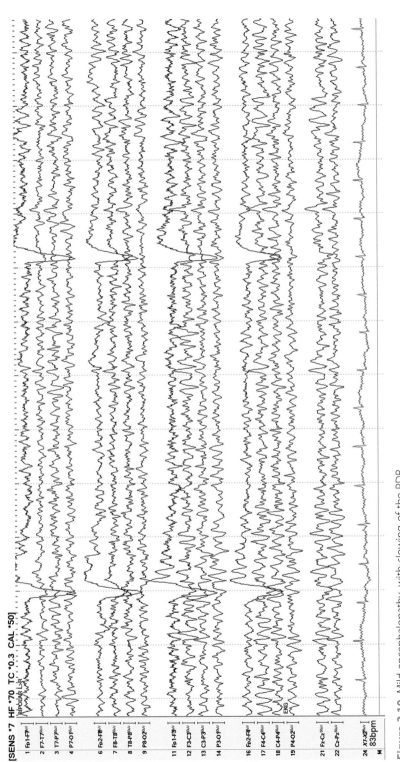

Figure 3.10 Mild encephalopathy, with slowing of the PDR.

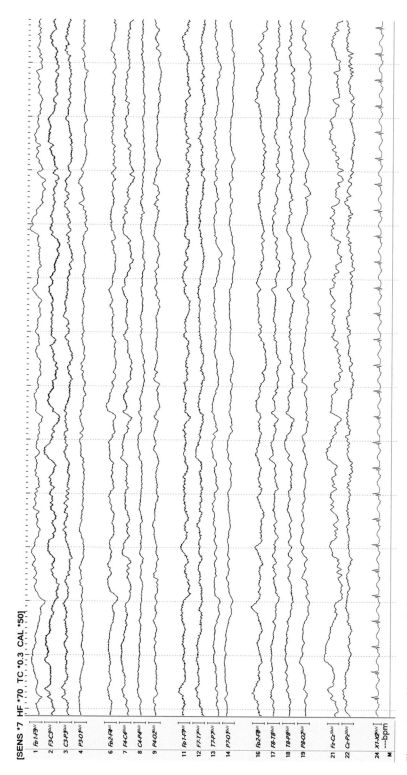

Figure 3.11 Moderate encephalopathy, with loss of the PDR.

Qualitative Grading of Encephalopathy

The severity of encephalopathy (global cerebral dysfunction) can be estimated based on the background. The key features are generalized slowing, loss of PDR, and, subsequently, loss of reactivity (either to external stimulus or state changes) with increasing severity.

- *Mild encephalopathy* is characterized by *slowing of the PDR* (8 Hz or less), excess slow activity in other areas, loss of normal organization (neatness of the EEG), and even the emergence of background discontinuity. Figure 3.10 shows mild encephalopathy.
- *Moderate encephalopathy* is characterized by complete *loss of the PDR*. The degree of generalized slowing increases, but EEG-R is still present. Stimulus induced (SI) or state dependent rhythmic or periodic patterns may also occur. Figure 3.11 shows moderate encephalopathy.
- *Severe encephalopathy* is characterized by *loss of reactivity*. The background is often (not always) discontinuous, with burst suppression or complete suppression. Rarely, continuous but unreactive patterns such as alpha coma or spindle coma occur.

Reversal of these trends suggests electrographic improvement, but not necessarily clinical improvement, which may be delayed. Furthermore, estimates of encephalopathy severity should not be confused with prognostication, as most EEG features are not specific to an etiology (e.g., EEG of anesthetic coma may be indistinguishable from hypoxic ischemic brain injury–both severe encephalopathies but with distinctly different prognoses) [6].

Finally, always correlate your EEG findings with the history, examination, laboratory, and neuroimaging results. Ask yourself: *How well do the EEG findings fit with the rest of the clinical presentation?*

Unexpected or discordant findings should arouse the reader's suspicion for an alternative explanation. Always reference the EEG report and, if in doubt, discuss your findings with an experienced reader.

References

1. Hirsch LJ, Fong MW, Leitinger M, et al. American Clinical Neurophysiology Society's Standardized Critical Care EEG Terminology: 2021 version. *Journal of Clinical Neurophysiology.* 2021 Jan 1;38(1):1–29.
2. Admiraal MM, Van Rootselaar AF, Horn J. International consensus on EEG reactivity testing after cardiac arrest: Towards standardization. *Resuscitation.* 2018 Oct 1;131:36–41.
3. Azabou E, Navarro V, Kubis N, et al. Value and mechanisms of EEG reactivity in the prognosis of patients with impaired consciousness: A systematic review. *Critical Care.* 2018 Dec;22(1):1–5.
4. Benghanem S, Paul M, Charpentier J, et al. Value of EEG reactivity for prediction of neurologic outcome after cardiac arrest: Insights from the Parisian registry. *Resuscitation.* 2019 Sep 1;142:168–74.
5. Admiraal MM, van Rootselaar AF, Hofmeijer J, et al. Electroencephalographic reactivity as predictor of neurological outcome in postanoxic coma: A multicenter prospective cohort study. *Annals of Neurology.* 2019 Jul;86(1):17–27.
6. Zafar S, Doria J, Karceski S. Should we standardize the EEG classification of mild, moderate, and severe cerebral dysfunction? *Epilepsy & Behavior: E&B.* 2020 Nov 1;112:107332.

Introduction

Recognizing Artifacts and Medication Effects

- What are artifacts?
- Internal artifacts
- External artifacts
- Common medication effects

- EEG patterns of intravenous anesthesia
- EEG patterns of inhalational anesthesia

What Are Artifacts?

Artifacts are waves detected by the EEG electrodes that originate outside the brain. Their source may be physiological (i.e., arising from other body organs – *internal artifacts*), or non-physiological (i.e., factors in the surrounding environment – *external artifacts*).

Artifacts are important to recognize as they can mimic abnormal waves or obscure the EEG. As mentioned earlier, busy acute care environments make the recording prone to contamination with artifacts. Potentially, any external or internal, electronic or mechanical device can generate artifact, and it is not always possible to safely move or switch off these devices to eliminate artifact. Therefore, the reader must learn to recognize artifacts.

Fortunately for the reader, external causes (e.g., humming of an infusion pump) may be time-locked to the artifact source and easily recognized at the bedside.

Therefore, if you identify artifact on EEG, carefully scan the bedside for potential sources. Some common ones are described here.

Common internal artifacts:

1. Ocular (eye movement)
2. Glossokinetic (tongue movement)
3. Cardiac (ECG artifact)
4. Myogenic (muscle artifact)
5. Skin (sweat sway artifact)

Common external artifacts:

1. Electrodes (including 60 Hz artifact)
2. Ventilator
3. Suctioning
4. Bed percussion
5. Chest compressions
6. Devices.

Internal Artifacts

Ocular (Eye) Artifacts

The globe behaves as a dipole, the cornea being positive and the retina relatively negative. In a standard electrode array (10–20 system) the frontopolar electrodes (Fp) are located above the eye and the frontal electrodes (F) beside it; therefore, vertical eye movements cause ocular artifact in the frontopolar electrodes (Fp1/2) and horizontal eye movements cause artifact in the frontal (F7/8) electrodes.

Movements generating ocular artifact include blinks, eye flutter, vertical eye movements, and horizontal eye movements (including nystagmus).

These are easily recognized at the bedside and correlated with the EEG. Carefully observe the patient's eyes:

(a) **Eyelid blink.** The cornea rolls upwards with closure of the eyelids; this is *Bell's phenomenon*. It results in a large downward (positive) deflection in the frontopolar channels (Fp1/2). Eye opening has an opposite effect with a large upward (negative) deflection in the frontopolar channels. Figure 4.1 shows eyelid blink and opening.

(b) **Eyelid flutter.** Rapid blinking or eye fluttering results in a bilateral, rhythmic, high amplitude, slow wave artifact maximal in the frontopolar channels. It may mimic generalized rhythmic delta activity (GRDA). Figure 4.2 shows eyelid flutter.

(c) **Eye movements:**
   (i) *Vertical movements.* Upward eye movement results in downward (positive) deflections in the frontopolar channels (Fp 1/2) while downward eye movements have an opposite effect. Vertical nystagmus (ocular bobbing) results in sharp upward (negative) deflections corresponding to the rapid down phase with slow returns. Figure 4.3 shows vertical eye movements.
   (ii) *Horizontal movements.* When the eyes turn to the left, there is leftward movement of the cornea resulting in downward (positive) deflections in the F7 channel. When they turn to the right, there is downward (positive) deflection in the F8 channel. Often, a small artifactual spike (lateral rectus spike) may precede the lateral eye movements artifact. Slow horizontal eye movements are normal during drowsiness and

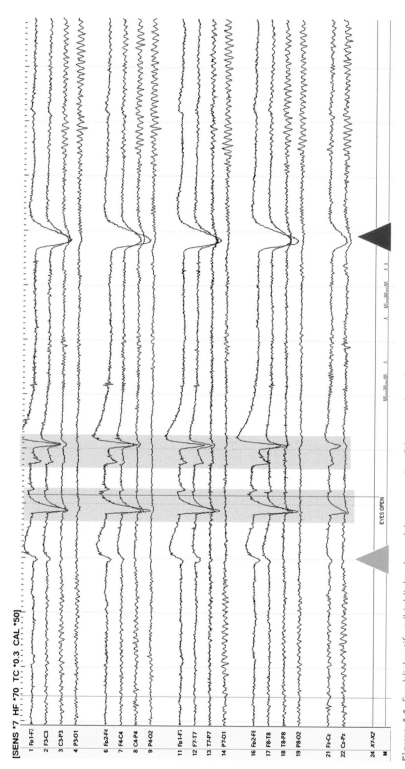

Figure 4.1 Eye blink artifact (highlighted purple), eye opening (blue arrow), and eye closure (red arrow).

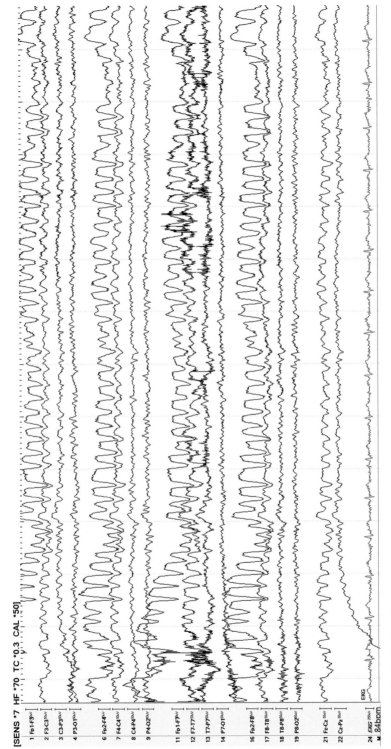

Figure 4.2 Eyelid flutter artifact.

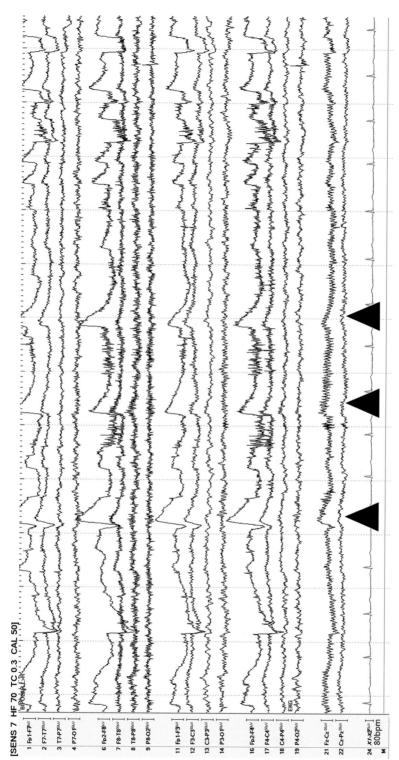

Figure 4.3 Vertical eye movement artifacts (black arrows).

result in sinusoidal waveforms at F7/F8. Lateral nystagmus may also cause similar waveforms in these channels. Figure 4.4 shows horizontal eye movements.

Glossokinetic (Tongue) Artifact

The tip of the tongue is negatively charged relative to its base. Tongue movements such as speaking, swallowing, or sipping lead to prominent bursts of high amplitude, frontal predominant, generalized delta frequency artifact with a wide field and often a squared-off shape. There is usually superimposed muscle artifact. Glossokinetic artifact may also mimic GRDA. Figure 4.5 shows glossokinetic artifact.

Cardiac Artifacts

Electrical signals and pulsations of the heart cause artifact that is time-locked to the QRS complex. Irregular heart rhythms may lead to irregular appearing artifact. Common types include ECG artifact, pulse artifact, and cardioballistic artifact.

a) **ECG artifact** appears as narrow periodic spikes corresponding to the QRS complex. It may be generalized or lateralized. It is common in those with shorter, thicker necks. ECG artifact mimics periodic discharges. Figure 4.6 shows ECG artifact.

b) **Pulse artifact** results from placing an electrode over a pulsating artery. This creates a focal, rhythmic, rounded artifact that is time-locked to the QRS complex and is restricted to one electrode, which may have high impedances. Central and temporal channels are commonly affected, and the artifact mimics rhythmic focal slowing. Figure 4.7 shows pulse artifact.

c) **Cardioballistic artifact** results from mechanical pulsations of the heart. It appears as a diffuse, periodic, slow wave artifact that is time-locked to the QRS complex. This is common in thin patients; it may be exaggerated in the setting of a left ventricular assist device (LVAD). It can also be seen after cardiac arrest with diffuse hypoxic ischemic brain injury. Figure 4.8 shows cardioballistic artifact.

Myogenic Artifact (EMG)

Scalp muscle activity manifests as high amplitude, very fast, and spiky artifact that may obscure the recording. Usually, the midline channels (Fz-Cz and Cz-Pz) are relatively free of this artifact since the scalp midline lacks underlying muscle. These channels provide the reader a window to observe the underlying EEG in cases of excessive muscle artifact. High frequency filters (HFF) may also be helpful. Jaw clenching worsens the artifact, and jaw relaxation reduces it. Figure 4.9 shows excessive muscle artifact.

Occasionally, neuromuscular blockade may be necessary to identify underlying EEG activity such as in postanoxic myoclonus [1].

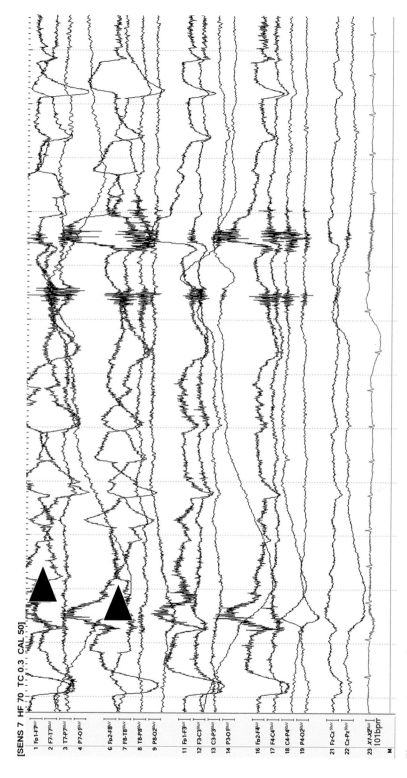

Figure 4.4 Horizontal eye movement artifacts (black arrows).

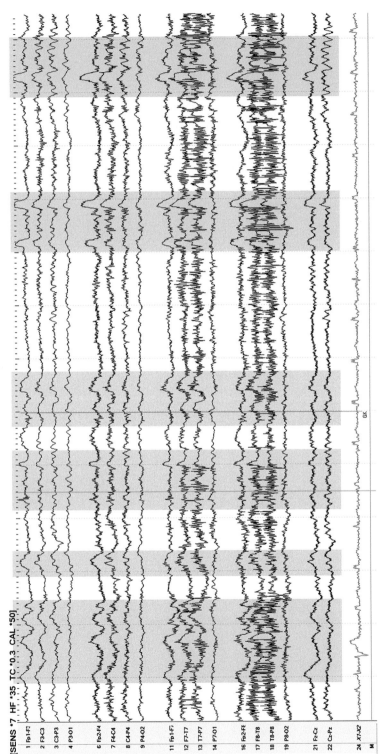

Figure 4.5 Glossokinetic artifact (highlighted purple).

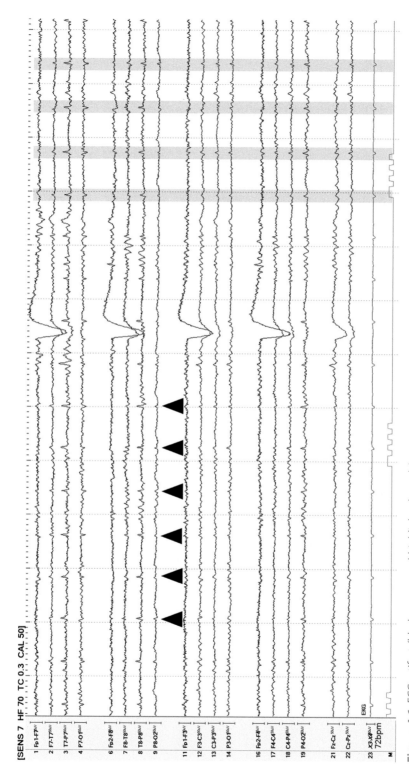

[SENS 7 HF 70 TC 0.3 CAL 50]

1 Fp1-F7
2 F7-T7
3 T7-P7
4 P7-O1

6 Fp2-F8
7 F8-T8
8 T8-P8
9 P8-O2

11 Fp1-F3
12 F3-C3
13 C3-P3
14 P3-O1

16 Fp2-F4
17 F4-C4
18 C4-P4
19 P4-O2

21 Fz-Cz
22 Cz-Pz

23 X3-X4
72bpm

EKG

M

Figure 4.6 ECG artifact (black arrows, and highlighted purple).

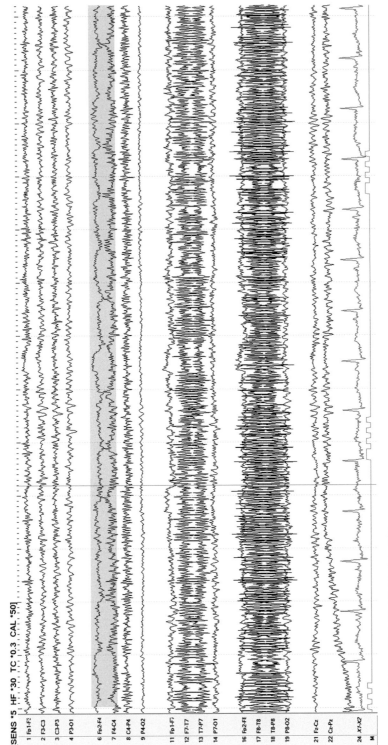

[SENS *5 HF *30 TC *0.3 CAL *50]

1 Fp1-F3
2 F3-C3
3 C3-P3
4 P3-O1

6 Fp2-F4
7 F4-C4
8 C4-P4
9 P4-O2

11 Fp1-F7
12 F7-T7
13 T7-P7
14 P7-O1

16 Fp2-F8
17 F8-T8
18 T8-P8
19 P8-O2

21 Fz-Cz
22 Cz-Pz

24 X1-X2

M

Figure 4.7 Pulse artifact (highlighted purple).

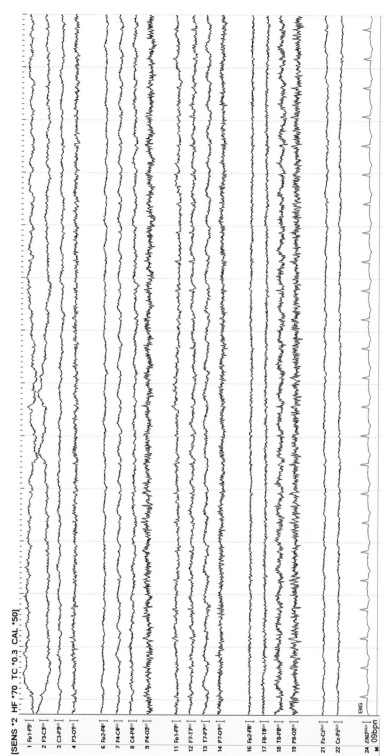

Figure 4.8 Cardioballistic artifact.

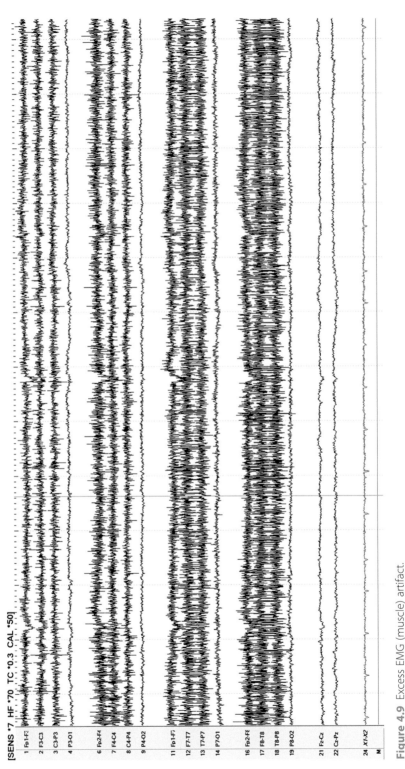

Figure 4.9 Excess EMG (muscle) artifact.

Chewing artifact has a generalized, regular, or clonic appearance. Figure 4.10 shows chewing artifact.

Skin (Sweat) Artifact

Sweating skin results in salt bridges forming between electrodes. This can cause a slow irregular artifact (sway) that may affect single or multiple channels.

Diffuse sweat artifact can mimic GRDA. Wiping moisture off the scalp resolves it. Figure 4.11 shows "sweat sway" artifact.

External Artifacts

Electrode Artifact

A change in impedance from the loss of electrode contact causes artifact. This can have a sharp, rhythmic, or periodic appearance that may mimic epileptiform discharges or even electrographic seizures. *Unlike cerebral activity, artifact is restricted to the problem electrode and lacks a physiological field.*

60 Hz artifact: Alternating current sources (e.g., electronic equipment) may manifest in poorly applied electrodes and cause 60 Hz artifact. Unusual patterns may result when it affects multiple channels simultaneously. It can be easily identified by switching off the 60 Hz notch filter. Reapplying loose electrodes and moving away adjacent electronic devices from the patient's head improves it. (Please note that this 60 Hz artifact applies to North America, but many other regions of the world including most of the Eastern hemisphere use 50 Hz alternating current and therefore have a **50 Hz artifact** instead of 60 Hz.)

Figure 4.12 shows electrode "pop" artifact (no field); Figure 4.13 shows 60 Hz electrode artifact before (a) and after (b) the 60 Hz notch filter is switched off.

Ventilator Artifact

Typically, this is a generalized, periodic, slow wave artifact with temporal or occipital predominance that occurs at the respiratory rate. Rarely, it may occur at twice the respiratory rate (inhalation and exhalation). It may also have a sharp, complex, or irregular appearance. It results from both respiratory movements themselves, as well as condensation in the ventilator tubing (rattle). Figure 4.14 shows ventilator artifact.

- A specific type of rhythmic ventilator artifact occurs with oscillations of *water trapped in the endotracheal tube (rattle)*. This causes frontal predominant rhythmic bursts of alpha, theta, or beta frequency that may mimic seizures. Suctioning the ET tube corrects the artifact. Figure 4.15 shows artifact resulting from water trapped in the ET tube.

Suctioning

Suctioning typically creates semi-rhythmic, irregular, theta and delta activity. Waveforms may be squared-off, and they usually have an abrupt start and finish.

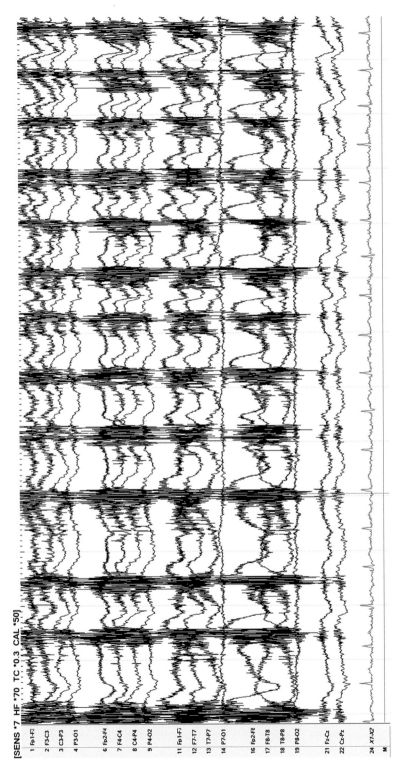

Figure 4.10 Chewing artifact.

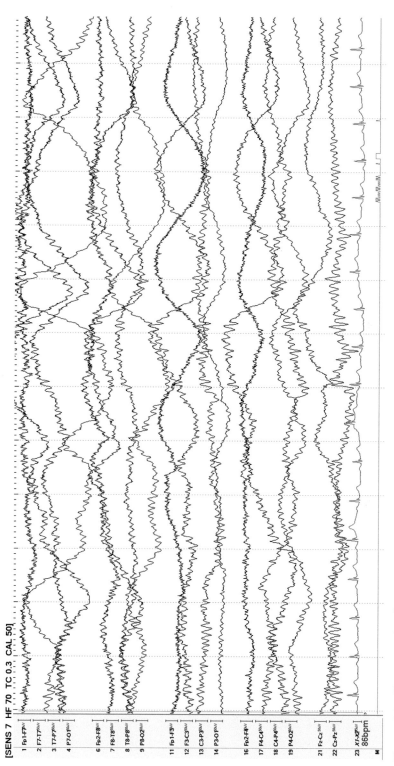

Figure 4.11 "Sweat sway" artifact.

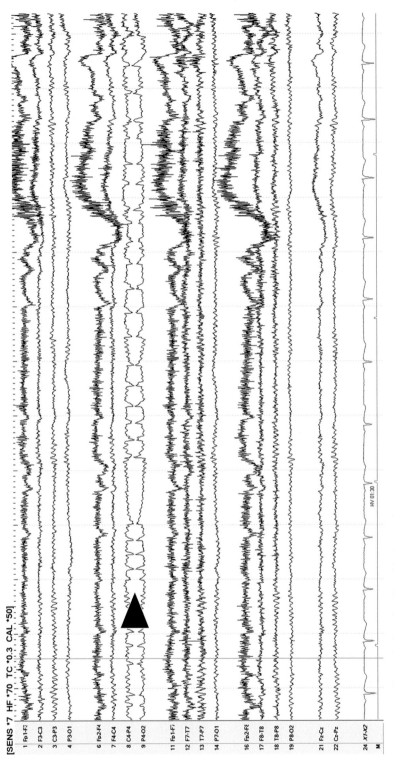

[SENS *7 HF *70 TC *0.3 CAL *50]

1 Fp1-F3
2 F3-C3
3 C3-P3
4 P3-O1

6 Fp2-F4
7 F4-C4
8 C4-P4
9 P4-O2

11 Fp1-F7
12 F7-T7
13 T7-P7
14 P7-O1

16 Fp2-F8
17 F8-T8
18 T8-P8
19 P8-O2

21 Fz-Cz
22 Cz-Pz

24 X1-X2
M

HV 01:30

Figure 4.12 Electrode "pop" artifact (black arrow).

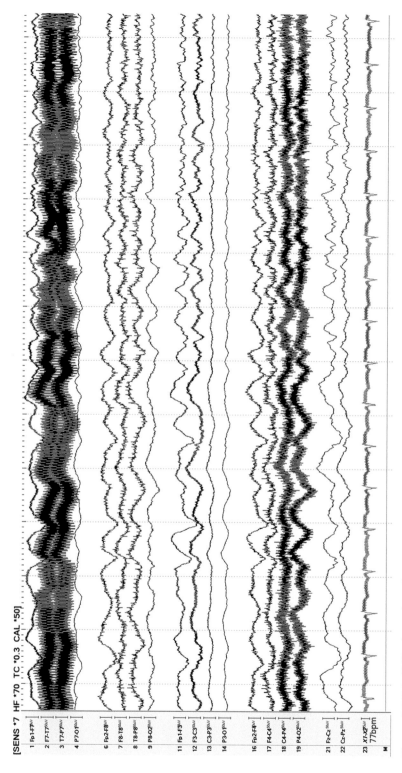

[SENS *7 HF *70 TC *0.3 CAL *50]

1 Fp1-F7(μV)
2 F7-T7(μV)
3 T7-P7(μV)
4 P7-O1(μV)

6 Fp2-F8(μV)
7 F8-T8(μV)
8 T8-P8(μV)
9 P8-O2(μV)

11 Fp1-F3(μV)
12 F3-C3(μV)
13 C3-P3(μV)
14 P3-O1(μV)

16 Fp2-F4(μV)
17 F4-C4(μV)
18 C4-P4(μV)
19 P4-O2(μV)

21 Fz-Cz(μV)
22 Cz-Pz(μV)

23 X1-X2(μV)
77bpm

M

Figure 4.13(a) 60 Hz electrode artifact most prominent at T7, P4.

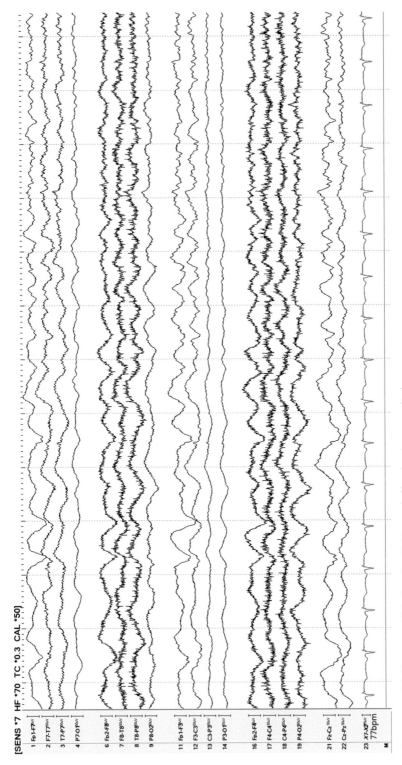

[SENS *7   HF *70   TC *0.3   CAL *50]

1 Fp1-F7(50uV)
2 F7-T7(50uV)
3 T7-P7(50uV)
4 P7-O1(50uV)

6 Fp2-F8(50uV)
7 F8-T8(50uV)
8 T8-P8(50uV)
9 P8-O2(50uV)

11 Fp1-F3(50uV)
12 F3-C3(50uV)
13 C3-P3(50uV)
14 P3-O1(50uV)

16 Fp2-F4(50uV)
17 F4-C4(50uV)
18 C4-P4(50uV)
19 P4-O2(50uV)

21 Fz-Cz(50uV)
22 Cz-Pz(50uV)

23 X1-X2(50uV)
77bpm

M

Figure 4.13(b) The same EEG after the 60 Hz notch filter has been applied.

[SENS *7 HF *70 TC *0.3 CAL *50]

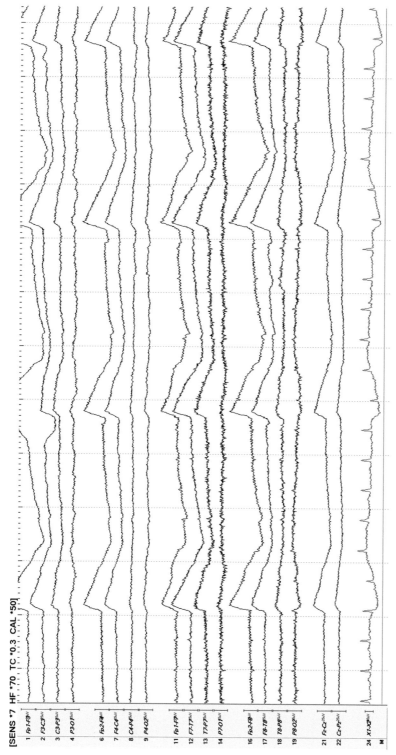

Figure 4.14 Ventilator movement artifact.

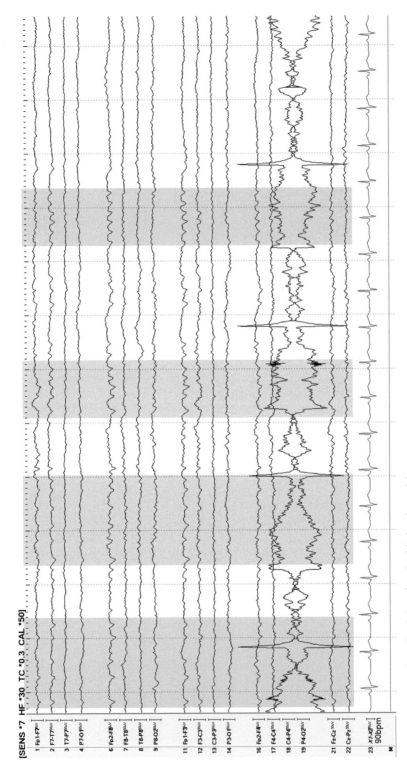

[SENS *7 HF *30 TC *0.3 CAL *50]

1 Fp1-F7^{>AV}
2 F7-T7^{>AV}
3 T7-P7^{>AV}
4 P7-O1^{>AV}

6 Fp2-F8^{>AV}
7 F8-T8^{>AV}
8 T8-P8^{>AV}
9 P8-O2^{>AV}

11 Fp1-F3^{>AV}
12 F3-C3^{>AV}
13 C3-P3^{>AV}
14 P3-O1^{>AV}

16 Fp2-F4^{>AV}
17 F4-C4^{>AV}
18 C4-P4^{>AV}
19 P4-O2^{>AV}

21 Fz-Cz^{>AV}
22 Cz-Pz^{>AV}

23 X1-X2^{>AV}
90bpm

M

Figure 4.15 Ventilator "rattle" artifact (highlighted purple).

Bed Percussion

This typically creates posterior predominant low amplitude rhythmic artifact that may begin in the theta range and terminate with faster frequencies. It may also spread in location with patient movement, mimicking electrographic seizures. Figure 4.16 shows bed percussion artifact.

Chest Compressions and Sternal Rubs

These create posterior predominant high amplitude rhythmic artifact.

External Medical Devices

Devices such as extracorporeal membrane oxygenation (ECMO), continuous veno-venous hemofiltration (CVVH), and hemodialysis (HD) may produce unusual rhythmic artifacts.

Again, these sources are recognizable at the bedside [2].

Common Medication Effects

Many commonly used medications are associated with EEG changes.

These include excess alpha and beta activity, theta and delta slowing, epileptiform abnormalities, and rhythmic or periodic patterns that may represent electrographic seizures or status epilepticus. These effects are common in the elderly, in those with cognitive impairment, and in those with renal dysfunction. Drug effects are typically generalized and symmetrical; asymmetry may suggest an underlying lesion.

Excess alpha and beta activity. *Barbiturates* and *benzodiazepines* produce excess generalized or frontally maximal beta activity. Alcohol withdrawal, central nervous system stimulants (cocaine, amphetamines, methylphenidate), and tricyclic antidepressants may also cause excess alpha and beta activity. Figure 4.17 shows excess beta activity.

Theta and delta slowing may be associated with toxicity from *antiseizure medications (ASMs)* such as phenytoin, carbamazepine, carbamazepine (10,11) epoxide, and valproate among other causes. Clozapine, tricyclic antidepressants, and lithium may also diffusely enhance theta and delta slowing in excess.

Spikes/sharp waves may be seen with *psychiatric medications* such as bupropion, clozapine, lithium, phenothiazines (e.g., chlorpromazine, fluphenazine, prochlorperazine), selective serotonin reuptake inhibitors, and tricyclic antidepressants. These are more likely seen at toxic doses. Reduction of antiseizure medications may also augment epileptic discharges. Clinical or electrographic seizures may be precipitated. Figure 4.18 shows a spike associated with clozapine.

Rhythmic and periodic patterns (RPPs), including those representing seizures and/or status epilepticus, may occur with toxicity from certain medications. Common patterns include *generalized periodic discharges (GPDs) with*

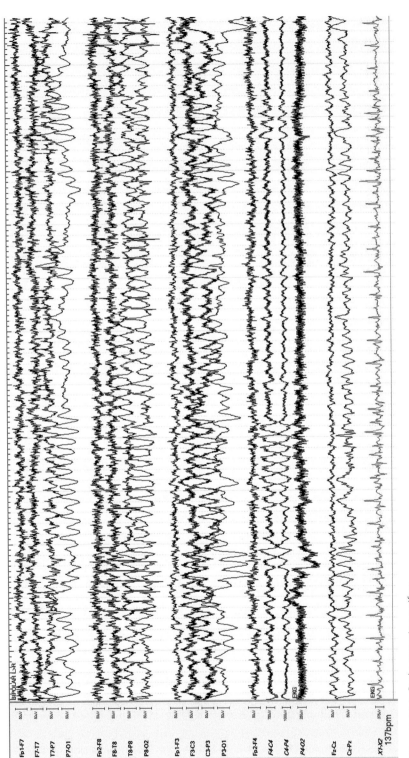

Figure 4.16 Bed percussion artifact.

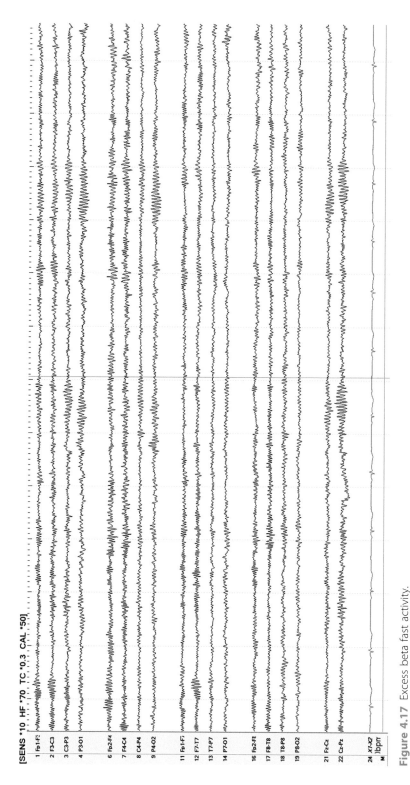

Figure 4.17 Excess beta fast activity.

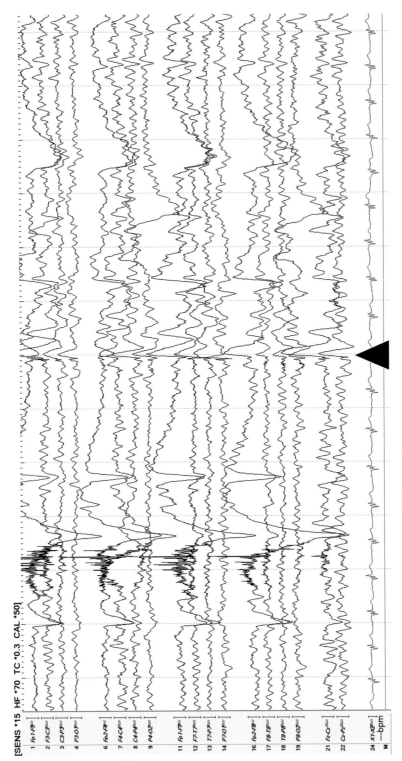

[SENS *15   HF *70   TC *0.3   CAL *50]

1	Fp1-F3⁽ᴬᵛ⁾
2	F3-C3⁽ᴬᵛ⁾
3	C3-P3⁽ᴬᵛ⁾
4	P3-O1⁽ᴬᵛ⁾
6	Fp2-F4⁽ᴬᵛ⁾
7	F4-C4⁽ᴬᵛ⁾
8	C4-P4⁽ᴬᵛ⁾
9	P4-O2⁽ᴬᵛ⁾
11	Fp1-F7⁽ᴬᵛ⁾
12	F7-T7⁽ᴬᵛ⁾
13	T7-P7⁽ᴬᵛ⁾
14	P7-O1⁽ᴬᵛ⁾
16	Fp2-F8⁽ᴬᵛ⁾
17	F8-T8⁽ᴬᵛ⁾
18	T8-P8⁽ᴬᵛ⁾
19	P8-O2⁽ᴬᵛ⁾
21	Fz-Cz⁽ᴬᵛ⁾
22	Cz-Pz⁽ᴬᵛ⁾
24	X1-X2⁽ᴬᵛ⁾
M	---bpm

Figure 4.18 Spike associated with clozapine use (black arrow).

triphasic morphology (also known as triphasic waves) and *generalized rhythmic delta activity (GRDA)*.

Common culprits include *antibiotic associated encephalopathy* (especially *cefepime*), *chemotherapeutics* (bevacizumab, cyclosporine, cytarabine, doxorubicin, etoposide, ifosfamide, L-asparaginase, and vincristine), and *immune modulators* (tacrolimus). GPDs may also occur with toxicities/withdrawal of baclofen, levodopa, lithium, opiates, and pentobarbital. *Valproic acid associated hyperammonemic encephalopathy* is a less frequent cause [3,4].

Figure 4.19 shows GPDs with triphasic morphology (previously called triphasic waves) with cefepime (antibiotic) associated encephalopathy.

EEG Patterns with Intravenous Anesthesia

Propofol enhances the GABA-A receptor mediated inhibition of the cortex, thalamus, and brainstem. Sedation with propofol is associated with diffuse excess alpha and/or beta activity. High amplitude delta slowing may occur when propofol is administered as a bolus for induction. Unconsciousness is associated with low amplitude, delta slowing with nearly continuous *frontal alpha range spindle activity* (resembling sleep spindles). Further depth of anesthesia (medically induced coma) results in burst suppression, followed by complete suppression. Emergence from propofol anesthesia is characterized by a gradual return of faster frequencies.

Propofol infusions may also be associated with paradoxical excitation and rarely myoclonus [5]. Figure 4.20 shows propofol spindles.

Ketamine preferentially binds to the NMDA receptors (glutamate) on the inhibitory interneurons of the brain and spinal cord leading to neuronal excitation, resulting in increased cerebral metabolism and cortical blood flow. Disassociation, euphoria, and hallucinations are common at low doses. The EEG shows *excessive beta activity*. At higher doses, excitatory neurons are also blocked with loss of consciousness. Figure 4.21 shows ketamine effect.

Dexmedetomidine is a sedative and adjunct anesthetic commonly used in the ICU and ORs. It is a selective agonist of the presynaptic alpha-2 receptors of the locus coeruleus. Hyperpolarization of the locus coeruleus results in a loss of hypothalamic inhibition, triggering a non-rapid eye movement sleep-like state. Though sedated, the patient can be easily aroused and there is little risk of respiratory depression. EEG shows a pattern of *sleep spindles and semi-rhythmic high amplitude delta slowing* that closely resembles slow wave sleep. Figure 4.22 shows dexmedetomidine effect.

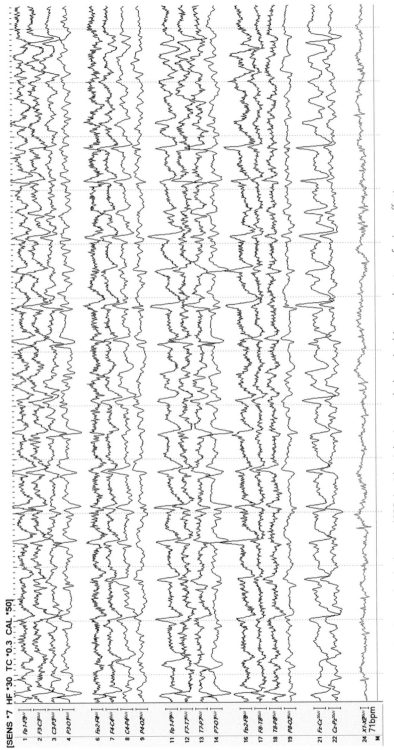

Figure 4.19 Generalized periodic discharges (GPDs) with triphasic morphology, in this case due to cefepime effect.

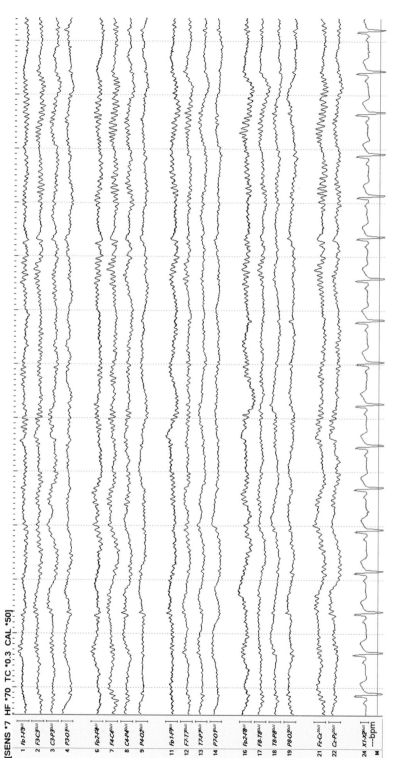

Figure 4.20 Propofol medication effect.

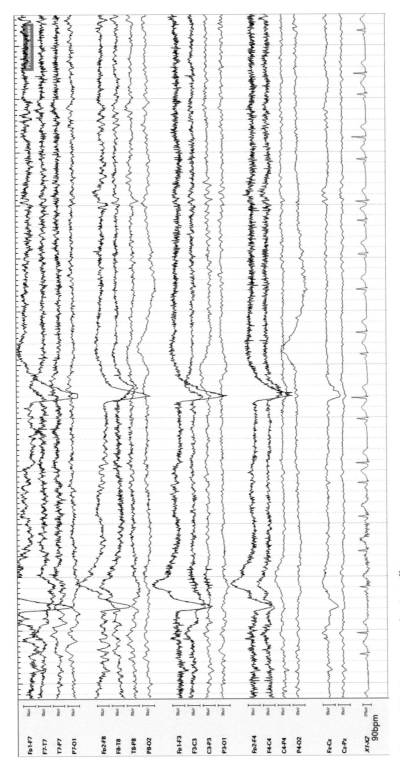

Figure 4.21 Ketamine medication effect.

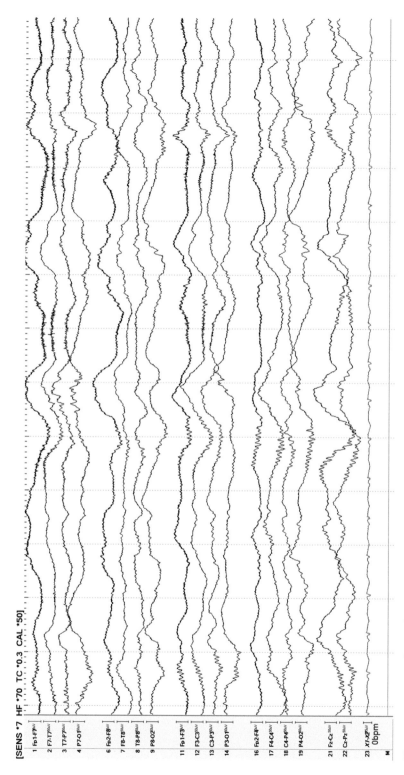

Figure 4.22 Dexmedetomidine medication effect.

EEG Patterns with Inhalational Anesthesia

Sevoflurane, isoflurane, and desflurane (ether derivatives) potentiate GABAergic inhibition among other actions to produce general anesthesia. At below minimum alveolar concentrations (MAC), the EEG shows delta slowing with bursts of alpha activity as with propofol. Maintenance of levels at or above MAC results in the emergence of theta activity, which suggests profound unconsciousness and immobility. Burst suppression or complete suppression is seen at higher doses.

Nitrous oxide is an adjunct anesthetic that is typically associated with excess fast activity. Transition to high flow nitrous oxide after maintenance with an ether anesthetic may result in transient, high amplitude, generalized delta slowing that eventually dissipates with return of excess fast activity [6].

References

1. Newey CR, Hornik A, Guerch M, Veripuram A, Yerram S, Ardelt A. The benefit of neuromuscular blockade in patients with postanoxic myoclonus otherwise obscuring continuous electroencephalography (CEEG). *Critical Care Research and Practice.* 2017 Feb 6;2017.
2. White DM, Van Cott CA. EEG artifacts in the intensive care unit setting. *American Journal of Electroneurodiagnostic Technology.* 2010 Mar 1;50(1):8–25.
3. Blume WT. Drug effects on EEG. *Journal of Clinical Neurophysiology.* 2006 Aug 1; 23(4):306–11.
4. Bhattacharyya S, Darby RR, Raibagkar P, Castro LN, Berkowitz AL. Antibiotic-associated encephalopathy. *Neurology.* 2016 Mar 8;86(10):963–71.
5. Hughes NJ, Lyons JB. Prolonged myoclonus and meningism following propofol. *Canadian Journal of Anaesthesia.* 1995 Aug 1;42(8):744–6.
6. Purdon PL, Sampson A, Pavone KJ, Brown EN. Clinical electroencephalography for anesthesiologists: Part I: Background and basic signatures. *Anesthesiology.* 2015 Oct;123(4):937–60.

Chapter | **Epileptiform Discharges, Seizures, and Status Epilepticus**

5

- Define epileptiform discharge
- Define seizure
- Define status epilepticus
- Electrographic criteria for seizures
- Electrographic criteria for status epilepticus

- Brief potentially ictal rhythmic discharges (BIRDs)
- Refractory status epilepticus
- Super-refractory status epilepticus

Arguably, the primary goal of continuous EEG monitoring in most cases is to diagnose seizures and status epilepticus that are not clinically obvious. Like clinical seizures, seizures on the EEG (electrographic seizures) can have a wide variety of appearances and implications. While status epilepticus is a well-defined and widely known neurological emergency, non-convulsive (subtle) status epilepticus remains an underdiagnosed cause of persistent unexplained encephalopathy or coma. Continuous EEG is essential for diagnosis and treatment.

Define Epileptiform Discharge

Epileptiform discharges are EEG transients (waves that come and go) that are typically sharp and have a specific morphology (see Chapter 3, Abnormal Waves). However, an epileptiform discharge ≠ *epileptic seizure!*

A seizure may be composed of many successive epileptiform discharges. It is not a perfect analogy, but it may help to think of the following example: *A single epileptiform discharge is to a seizure as a premature ventricular contraction (PVC) is to ventricular tachycardias.*

Epileptiform discharges can have various shapes, including:

- Spike: <70 ms from baseline to baseline
- Sharp waves: 70–200 ms from baseline to baseline
- Spike-wave: a spike with an "after going slow wave"

- Sharp-slow wave: a sharp with an "after going slow wave"
- Polyspikes: multiple successive spikes
- Paroxysmal fast activity: unexplained "buzz" of typically beta frequency activity.

Though they have different shapes, epileptiform discharges have similar implications: They indicate *cortical irritability* (sometimes termed cortical hyperexcitability) and confer *increased seizure RISK*.

All epileptiform discharges may be either *focal* (originating in a discrete area of the brain) or *generalized* (visible over the entire scalp at once). The type of epileptiform discharge may give clues as to the onset of a patient's seizures, which may help guide treatment. Figures 5.1 and 5.2 show examples of typical *focal* and *generalized* epileptiform discharges.

Some readers may use the term *"sharp transient."* This indicates that the transient lacks definite epileptiform morphology and that there is some ambiguity in its clinical implication. When in doubt, always speak directly to the electroencephalographer reporting your EEG.

Epileptiform discharges generally do not need to be treated or suppressed in and of themselves, though they may merit antiseizure medication (ASM) "prophylaxis" depending on the clinical context.

Define Seizure

Many definitions of seizure exist, but one common definition from the International League Against Epilepsy is *"a transient occurrence of signs and/or symptoms due to abnormal excessive or synchronous neuronal activity in the brain."* Many, but not all, seizures can be detected on EEG. When they are, they are known as *electrographic* or *electroclinical* seizures [1].

Define Status Epilepticus

Many definitions of status epilepticus exist, but colloquially this *"maximal expression of epilepsy"* entails prolonged, uncontrolled seizures or multiple successive seizures without return to baseline in between [2].

Status epilepticus involving clinically obvious seizures does *not* require EEG to diagnose, and treatment should *not* be delayed while waiting for EEG in these cases. However, CEEG is essential for the diagnosis and treatment of status epilepticus not causing obvious clinical signs or manifesting only with coma with or without additional subtle signs.

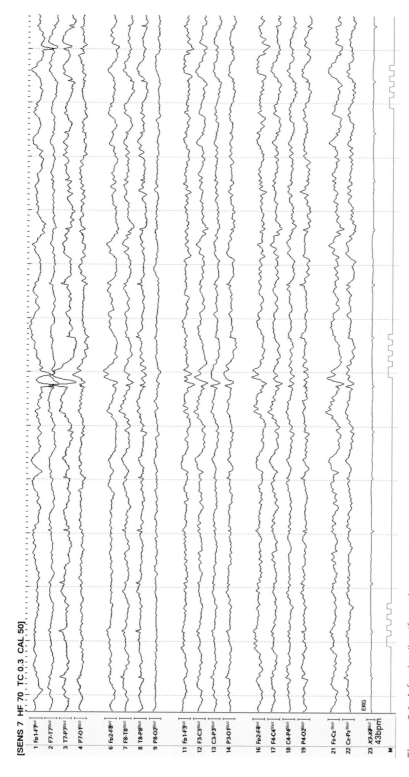

[SENS 7 HF 70 TC 0.3 CAL 50]

1 Fp1-F7
2 F7-T7
3 T7-P7
4 P7-O1

6 Fp2-F8
7 F8-T8
8 T8-P8
9 P8-O2

11 Fp1-F3
12 F3-C3
13 C3-P3
14 P3-O1

16 Fp2-F4
17 F4-C4
18 C4-P4
19 P4-O2

21 Fz-Cz
22 Cz-Pz

23 X3-X4
43bpm

EKG

Figure 5.1 A focal epileptiform sharp wave.

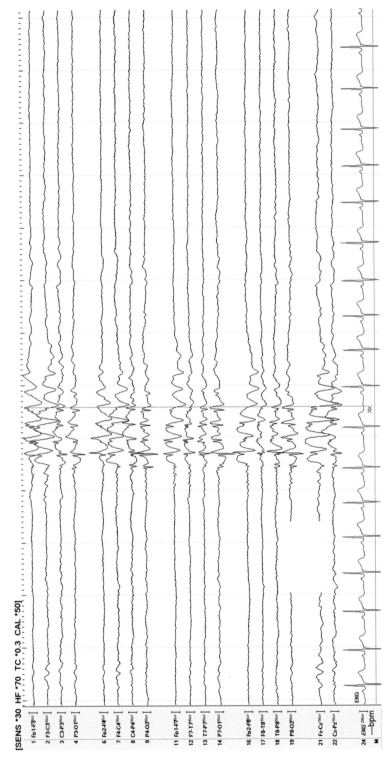

Figure 5.2 A brief run of generalized spike-wave discharges.

Electrographic Criteria for Seizures

According to the most recent iteration of the American Clinical Neurophysiology Society's (ACNS) Standardized Critical Care EEG Terminology [3], the following criteria for EEG diagnosis of seizure have been determined:

- **Electrographic seizure (ESz)**
  - This is a seizure diagnosed purely by electrographic criteria.
  - ACNS definitions:
    - "Epileptiform discharges averaging >2.5 Hz for ≥10 seconds (>25 discharges in 10 seconds)"
    - Any pattern with definite *evolution* and lasting ≥10 seconds; see Chapter 9 for a more in-depth explanation of *evolution*.
- **Electroclinical seizure (ECSz)**
  - This is a seizure that is diagnosed by both electrographic *and* clinical criteria, and does not necessarily meet all of the criteria for ESz.
  - ACNS definitions:
    - An abnormal EEG pattern with a "definite clinical correlate time-locked to the pattern (of any duration)"
    - Both "EEG *and* clinical improvement with a parenteral antiseizure medication."

Figure 5.3 shows an evolving electrographic seizure over three pages of EEG, (a) through (c).

Again, it bears repeating that not all seizures will be detected on scalp EEG. As many as two-thirds of subclinical or focal-aware seizures may go undetected on scalp EEG [4]! Always use your clinical judgement, and not EEG alone, when deciding whether to treat an episode concerning for seizure.

Seizures should typically be treated with ASMs. Chapter 11 covers the topic of treating seizures in greater depth.

Electrographic Criteria for Status Epilepticus

According to the 2021 ACNS Standardized Critical Care EEG Terminology [3], the following criteria for EEG diagnosis of status epilepticus have been determined, largely based on the earlier "Salzburg criteria," which are discussed further in Chapter 9:

- **Electrographic status epilepticus (ESE)**
  - This is status epilepticus diagnosed purely by electrographic criteria.
  - ACNS definition:
    - Electrographic seizure (ESz) ongoing for "≥10 continuous minutes (or for a total duration of ≥20% of any 60-minute period of recording)"
    - Any pattern with definite *evolution* and lasting ≥10 minutes; see Chapter 9 for a more in-depth explanation of *evolution*.

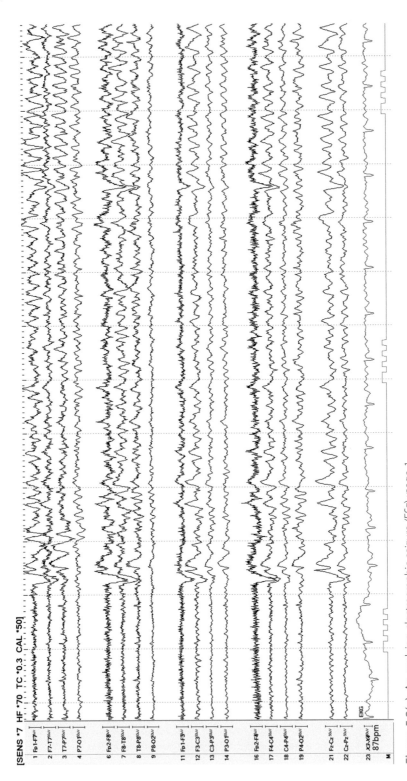

Figure 5.3(a) An evolving electrographic seizure (ESz), page 1.

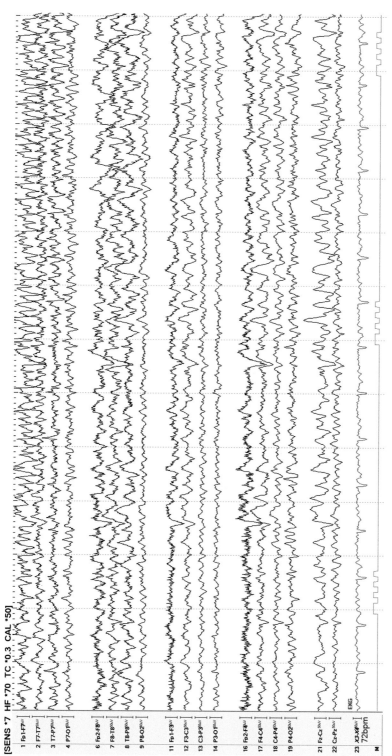

[SENS *7   HF *70   TC *0.3   CAL *50]

1 Fp1-F7⁵ᵘⱽ
2 F7-T7⁵ᵘⱽ
3 T7-P7⁵ᵘⱽ
4 P7-O1⁵ᵘⱽ

6 Fp2-F8⁵ᵘⱽ
7 F8-T8⁵ᵘⱽ
8 T8-P8⁵ᵘⱽ
9 P8-O2⁵ᵘⱽ

11 Fp1-F3⁵ᵘⱽ
12 F3-C3⁵ᵘⱽ
13 C3-P3⁵ᵘⱽ
14 P3-O1⁵ᵘⱽ

16 Fp2-F4⁵ᵘⱽ
17 F4-C4⁵ᵘⱽ
18 C4-P4⁵ᵘⱽ
19 P4-O2⁵ᵘⱽ

21 Fz-Cz⁵ᵘⱽ
22 Cz-Pz⁵ᵘⱽ
23 X3-X9⁵ᵘⱽ EKG
72bpm

M

Figure 5.3(b) An evolving electrographic seizure (ESz), page 2.

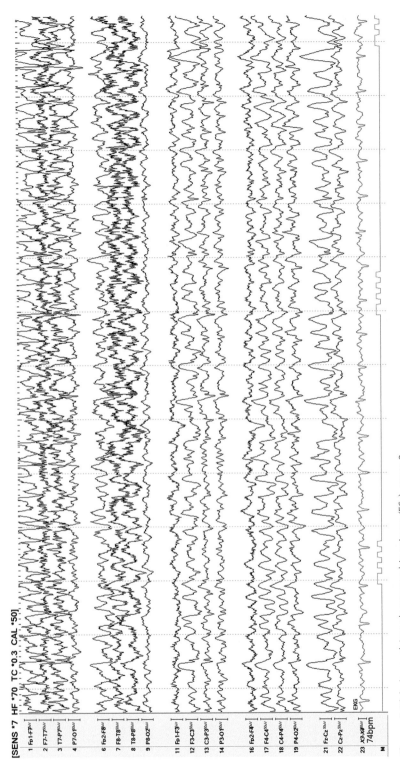

[SENS *7 HF *70 TC *0.3 CAL *50]

1 Fp1-F7
2 F7-T7
3 T7-P7
4 P7-O1

6 Fp2-F8
7 F8-T8
8 T8-P8
9 P8-O2

11 Fp1-F3
12 F3-C3
13 C3-P3
14 P3-O1

16 Fp2-F4
17 F4-C4
18 C4-P4
19 P4-O2

21 Fz-Cz
22 Cz-Pz

23 X3-X4
74bpm

EKG

M

Figure 5.3(c) An evolving electrographic seizure (ESz), page 3.

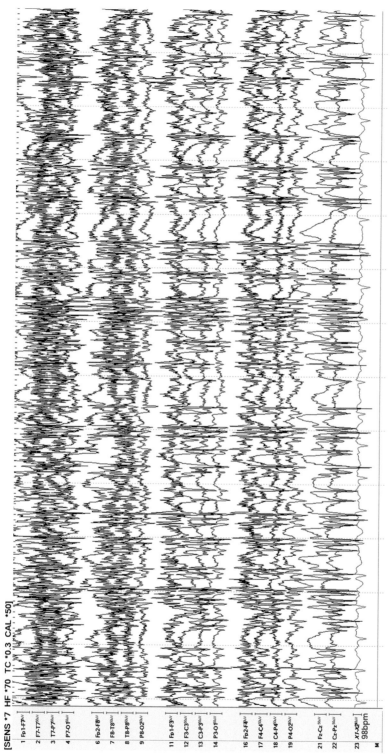

Figure 5.4 Electrographic status epilepticus (ESE).

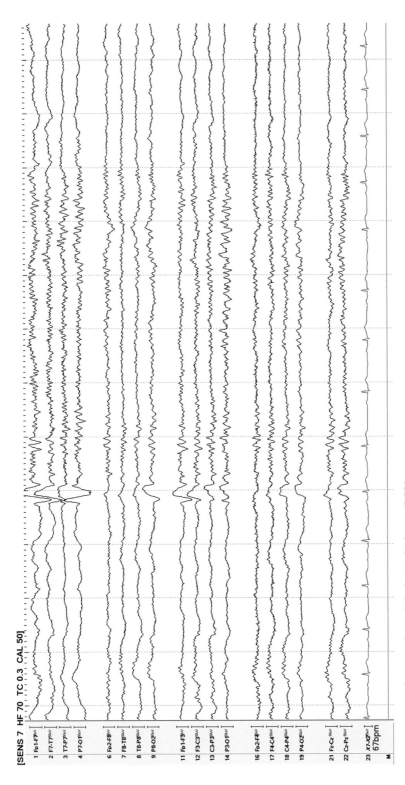

Figure 5.5 Brief potentially ictal rhythmic discharge (BIRD).

- **Electroclinical status epilepticus (ECSE)**
  - This is status epilepticus that is diagnosed by both electrographic *and* clinical criteria, and does not necessarily meet all of the criteria for ESE.
  - ACNS definition:
    - Electroclinical seizure activity (ECSz) ongoing for "$\geq$10 continuous minutes (or for a total duration of $\geq$20% of any 60-minute period of recording)."
    - For generalized tonic clonic convulsions (GTC) or secondarily generalized "bilateral tonic-clonic" convulsions (BTC), $\geq$5 minutes of ongoing seizure activity meets the criteria for ECSE.

Figure 5.4 shows an example of electrographic status epilepticus (ESE).

See Chapters 5 and 10 for more information on the ictal-interictal continuum (IIC) and the concept of "possible electroclinical status epilepticus." Chapter 9 covers the topic of treating status epilepticus in greater depth.

Brief Potentially Ictal Rhythmic Discharges (BIRDs)

By convention, and as defined by the ACNS above, when abnormal or *evolving* epileptiform discharges last *less than 10 seconds, and do NOT cause obvious clinical signs or symptoms*, this does NOT technically qualify as a seizure.

Until relatively recently, these EEG discharges did not have a proper name. Today, they are known as brief potentially ictal rhythmic discharges (BIRDs) [5–8], implying that they may (and often do) indicate high seizure risk, or even represent true seizure activity not readily detectable using scalp EEG. See Figure 5.5 for an example of a BIRD.

Refractory Status Epilepticus

When status epilepticus does not respond to an initial parenteral benzodiazepine medication and an additional ASM, it is considered *refractory* status epilepticus (RSE). This is typically treated with medically induced coma and is covered in more depth in Chapter 9.

Super-Refractory Status Epilepticus

When medically induced coma involving adequate doses of intravenous anesthetic agents does not suppress seizures and other epileptiform activity, it is considered to be *super-refractory* status epilepticus (SRSE). This topic, including management strategies, is covered in more detail through cases in Chapter 9.

References

1. Fisher RS, van Emde Boas W, Blume W, et al. Epileptic seizures and epilepsy: Definitions proposed by the International League Against Epilepsy (ILAE) and the International Bureau for Epilepsy (IBE). *Epilepsia*. 2005 Apr;46(4):470–2.

2. Trinka E, Kälviäinen R. 25 years of advances in the definition, classification and treatment of status epilepticus. *Seizure.* 2017 Jan;44:65–73.
3. Hirsch LJ, Fong MWK, Leitinger M, et al. American Clinical Neurophysiology Society's Standardized Critical Care EEG Terminology: 2021 version. *Journal of Clinical Neurophysiology.* 2021 Jan 1;38(1):1–29.
4. Casale MJ, Marcuse LV, Young JJ, et al. The sensitivity of scalp EEG at detecting seizures – a simultaneous scalp and stereo EEG study. *Journal of Clinical Neurophysiology.* 2022 Jan 1;39(1):78–84.
5. Yoo JY. BIRDs (brief potentially ictal rhythmic discharges) watching during EEG monitoring. *Frontiers in Neurology.* 2022 Aug 23;13:966480.
6. Yoo JY, Jetté N, Kwon CS, et al. Brief potentially ictal rhythmic discharges and paroxysmal fast activity as scalp electroencephalographic biomarkers of seizure activity and seizure onset zone. *Epilepsia.* 2021 Mar;62(3):742–51.
7. Yoo JY, Marcuse LV, Fields MC, et al. Brief potentially ictal rhythmic discharges [B(I)RDs] in noncritically ill adults. *Journal of Clinical Neurophysiology.* 2017 May;34(3):222–9.
8. Yoo JY, Rampal N, Petroff OA, et al. Brief potentially ictal rhythmic discharges in critically ill adults. *JAMA Neurology.* 2014 Apr;71(4):454–62.

Chapter 6

Rhythmic and Periodic Patterns (RPPs) and the Ictal-Interictal Continuum (IIC)

- Standardized EEG terminology
- Common types of RPPs
- Common causes of RPPs
- Differentiate distinct ictal from interictal patterns

- Markers of higher risk and pathogenesis
- Ictal-interictal continuum (IIC)
- Management of RPP and IIC pattern

Rhythmic and periodic patterns (RPPs) are frequently encountered in critical care settings and have a wide variety of clinical implications ranging from mundane to emergent. In many cases, the clinical implications of RPPs are uncertain, riding between seizure risk and ictal activity with the potential for neurological injury (frank seizures). This concept has been defined as the ictal-interictal continuum (IIC).

As the name suggests, an RPP is simply a pattern of discharges or waves occurring in a "rhythmic" or "periodic" pattern. In this context, "rhythmic" refers to a relatively regular rate with no intervening background, and "periodic" refers to a relatively regular rate with periods of intervening background between the discharges.

RPPs often stand out from the background and may appear alarming. Using this approach to bedside EEG reading, acute care providers can determine the level of risk that the pattern indicates, and, in consultation with a neurologist, the next steps in diagnosis and treatment.

Standardized EEG Terminology for RPPs

The following terminology is derived from the American Clinical Neurophysiology Society's 2021 Standardized Critical Care EEG terminology [1–3]:

First, the RPP is defined by the **laterality**:

- Generalized (G): pattern occurs symmetrically and synchronously in both hemispheres
- Lateralized (L): pattern occurs primarily in only one hemisphere (right or left)
- Bilateral independent (Bi): pattern occurs in both hemispheres, but not synchronously and usually at different rates.

Then, the RPP is defined by the **morphology** of the discharge or waves:

- Periodic discharges (PDs): abnormal discharges (often, but not always sharp or spiky in morphology), with a clear period of intervening background between them
- Rhythmic delta activity (RDA): rhythmic, usually monomorphic, slow (delta) waves occurring in runs
- Spike-wave or sharp-slow wave (SW): similar to PDs, but each discharge is clearly followed by a rhythmic after going slow wave.

The presence of **modifiers** can also be assessed:

- Superimposed fast activity (+F): each discharge is associated with overriding fast activity
- Superimposed spikes, sharp waves, or sharply contoured waveforms (+S): applies to RDA only, where there are intermixed spikes or sharp waves within the RDA (though not occurring in a regular pattern)
- Superimposed rhythmic delta activity (+R): applies to PDs only, where there is simultaneous rhythmic or quasi-rhythmic slow activity, though not occurring synchronously with the PDs.

Finally, the **rate** of the RPP must be determined:

- In general, a slower rate (e.g., <0.5–1 Hz) denotes a lower risk pattern and is more reassuring.
- In general, a higher rate (e.g., ≥1 Hz) denotes a higher risk pattern and higher risk for seizures (or the pattern may represent an atypical seizure, especially if associated with clinical manifestations such as motor activity).
- An RPP occurring at a rate ≥2.5 Hz for ≥10 seconds is considered electrographic seizure (ESz), and ≥10 minutes is considered electrographic status epilepticus (ESE).

There are many other minor characteristics that one can use to describe the RPP, but these are difficult to interpret at the bedside.

In many cases it can be difficult to decide between GPD+R, GSW, or GRDA+S for example, especially if a pattern is changing.

However, rather than dwelling on the specific name of the pattern, focusing on other factors such as frequency may be more important.

Additionally, those RPPs that may be difficult to differentiate as rhythmic or periodic may be preferably labelled as "periodic."

Common Types of RPPs

GRDA: generalized rhythmic delta activity. GRDA is the pattern least associated with seizure risk. It is a relatively nonspecific finding and can be seen with various diffuse encephalopathies, deep midline subcortical dysfunction, or (importantly) with increased intracranial pressure (Figure 6.1).

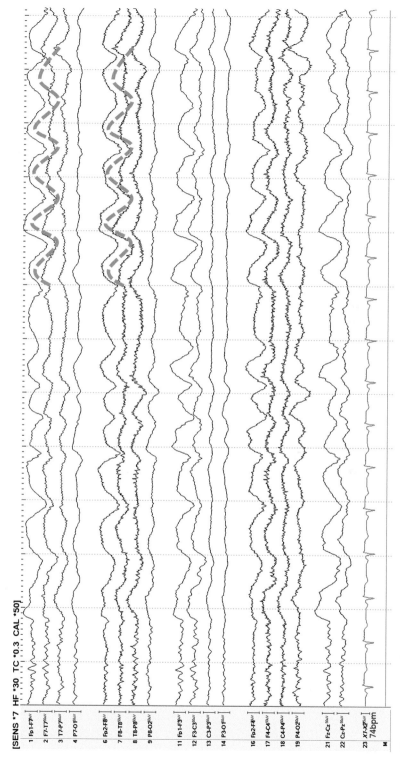

Figure 6.1 Generalized rhythmic delta activity (GRDA) at 1–1.5 Hz (highlighted with green line).

LRDA: lateralized rhythmic delta activity. LRDA, despite lacking sharp or spiky features, is considered an epileptiform "equivalent" and confers increased risk for seizures. This pattern can be seen in patients with known temporal lobe epilepsy (Figure 6.2).

GPDs (and **GSW**): generalized periodic discharges. GPDs vary widely in terms of their characteristics and implication based on several factors such as morphology, frequency, and etiology. This pattern indicates diffuse cortical hyperexcitability with increased seizure risk (Figure 6.3).

Triphasic waves (a.k.a. GPDs with triphasic morphology). These are a special type of GPDs classically associated with toxic metabolic disturbances such as hepatic encephalopathy, uremia, or infection. Their morphology is very particular, and they exhibit a characteristic "anterior–posterior lag." [4,5] (Figure 6.4).

LPDs (and **LSW**): lateralized periodic discharges. LPDs indicate focal cortical hyperexcitability and increased seizure risk from the region of the LPDs (Figure 6.5).

BiPDs: bilateral independent periodic discharges. BiPDs are similar to LPDs but occur independently in both hemispheres. They generally indicate a more diffuse or bilateral cerebral process and higher risk for seizure (Figure 6.6).

UiPDs: unilateral independent periodic discharges. These are similar to BiPDs, but the two independent foci are in the same hemisphere.

MfPDs: multifocal independent periodic discharges. These are similar to BiPDs, but with three or more distinct discharge foci.

Common Causes of RPPs

GRDA: Encephalopathy (nonspecific), deep midline subcortical dysfunction, increased intracranial pressure.

LRDA: Temporal lobe epilepsy, stroke, brain tumor, subdural hematoma, intracerebral hemorrhage, subarachnoid hemorrhage, focal encephalitis (infectious or autoimmune).

GPDs (and **GSW**): Encephalopathy (nonspecific), toxic metabolic disturbances, critical illness, multiorgan failure, generalized epilepsy syndromes, diffuse hypoxic ischemic brain injury, Creutzfeldt–Jacob disease.

GPDs with triphasic morphology: Encephalopathy (nonspecific), hepatic encephalopathy, uremia, infections, other toxic metabolic disturbances.

LPDs (and **LSW**): Stroke, encephalomalacia, brain tumor, subdural hematoma, subarachnoid hemorrhage, intracerebral hemorrhage, focal encephalitis (infectious or autoimmune).

BiPDs, UiPDs, MfPDs: Brain metastases, encephalitis, meningoencephalitis, multifocal intracranial hemorrhage.

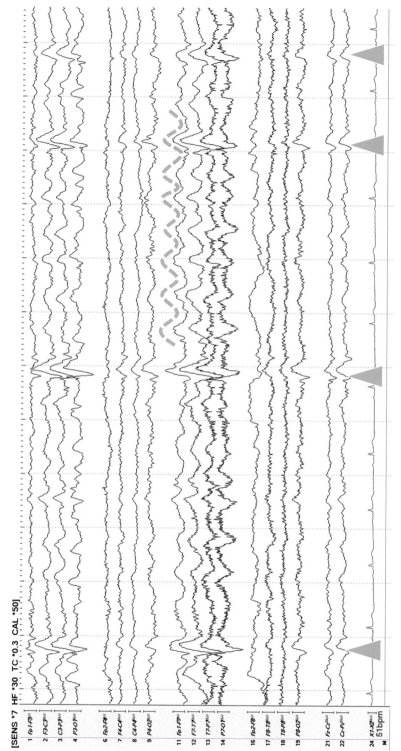

Figure 6.2 Lateralized rhythmic delta activity (LRDA) at 1.5–2 Hz (highlighted with blue line); in this case the intermixed sharp waves (blue arrows) make this LRDA "+S."

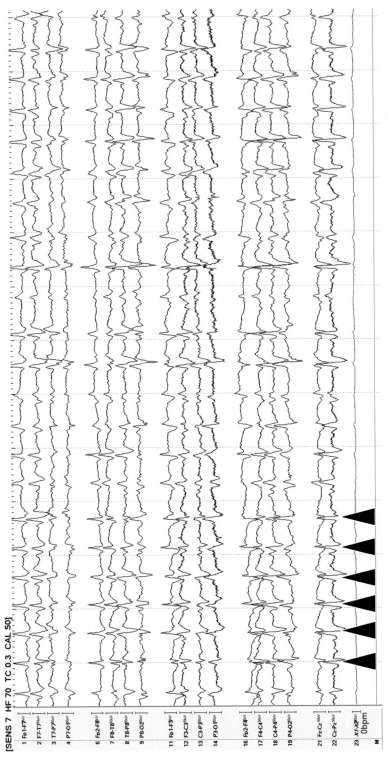

Figure 6.3 Generalized periodic discharges (GPDs) at 1.75–2 Hz (black arrows).

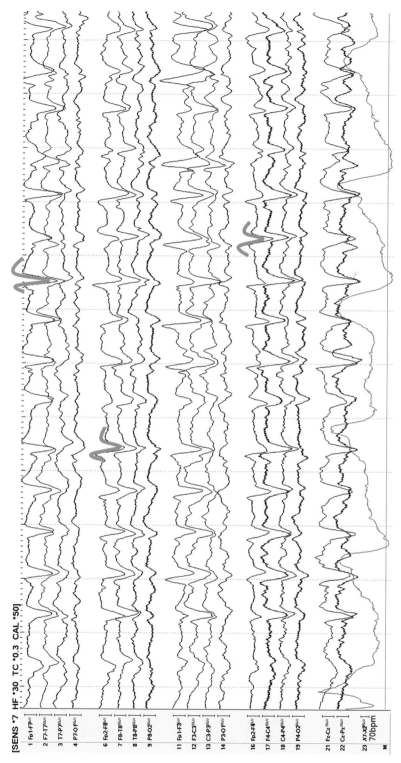

Figure 6.4 Generalized periodic discharges (GPDs) with triphasic morphology (emphasized with green lines) at 1–1.5 Hz, also known simply as periodic triphasic waves.

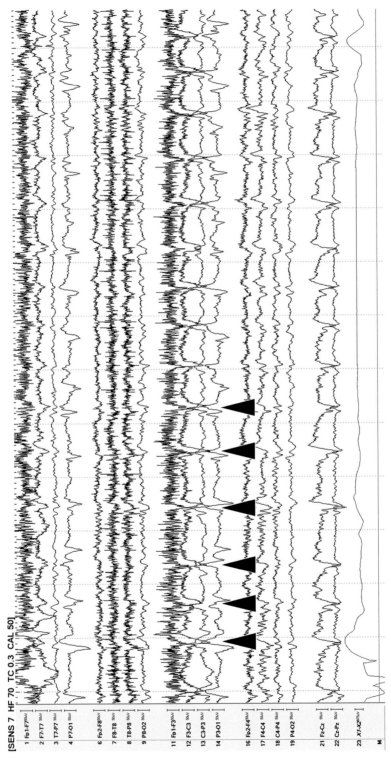

Figure 6.5 Lateralized periodic discharges (LPDs) at about 1 Hz (black arrows).

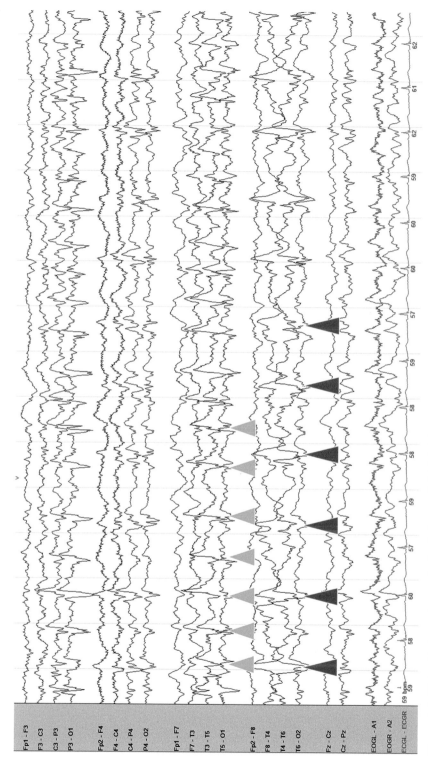

Figure 6.6 Bilateral independent periodic discharges (BiPDs); left hemisphere discharges marked with blue arrows, right hemisphere with red arrows.

Differentiate Distinct Ictal Patterns from Interictal Patterns

If a patient is awake and alert with no clinical symptoms while the pattern is ongoing, and no electrographic criteria for seizure are present, the pattern is clearly interictal.

If a patient has clear clinical symptoms associated with the abnormal EEG pattern, and there is both a clinical and EEG improvement with antiseizure medication, then the pattern is clearly ictal, and in fact is considered electroclinical seizure (ECSz) or electroclinical status epilepticus (ECSE) regardless of the frequency or other characteristics of the RPP.

However frequently the RPP occurs in an encephalopathy or in a comatose patient, often with other factors that confound the clinical assessment of mental status (e.g., sedative medications or CNS injuries). In these cases, when electrographic criteria for seizure are not met, things become less clear.

Markers of Higher Risk and Pathogenesis

In general, factors increasing the likelihood of seizure risk or actual clinical symptoms arising from the RPP include the following:

- **Frequency**: faster (higher frequency) > slower (lower frequency)
- **Modifiers**: RPPs with modifiers (such as superimposed fast activity) > plain RPPs
- **Voltage**: high voltage > very low voltage
- **Morphology**: spiky > sharp > blunt
- **Lack of stimulus or state dependence** i.e. present irrespective of stimulation or state change.

The more of these factors that are present, the more likely the pattern is to be indicative of high seizure risk, or even be a seizure itself (though not necessarily meeting formal electrographic criteria).

Ictal-Interictal Continuum (IIC)

A pattern that lies on the ictal-interictal continuum (IIC) does not meet formal criteria for a seizure, but nevertheless may be contributing to impaired alertness, causing neuronal injury, or otherwise causing clinical symptoms. A pattern on the IIC is essentially synonymous with "possible electroclinical status epilepticus," indicating that despite not meeting criteria for status epilepticus, the pattern may still represent a form of nonconvulsive status epilepticus with the potential for neurological injury [6–8].

Management of RPP and IIC Patterns

When an RPP is not clearly reassuring (e.g., classic triphasic waves), or not clearly benign (patient awake and alert with no symptoms), it is reasonable to consider a trial of intravenous antiseizure medication (ASM) and evaluate for electrographic (EEG) and clinical improvement.

For example, intravenous lorazepam or an intravenous load of an ASM such as levetiracetam, fosphenytoin, or lacosamide may be used in close consultation with a neurologist (or epileptologist).

In general:

GRDA: generally may not require treatment.

GPD with triphasic morphology: generally, initiation of treatment depends on the specific scenario and opinion of the treating neurologist.

LRDA, GPD, LPD, GSW, LSW: generally requires treatment with ASMs, but not necessarily suppression of the pattern.

Definite ictal features (i.e., evolution): generally require treatment *and* suppression of the abnormal pattern.

Clinic Scenarios

1. **Low risk**: A 40-year-old man with decompensated liver cirrhosis with occasional brief runs of blunted GPDs at 1 Hz with triphasic morphology. *This pattern does not necessarily require treatment with ASMs given it is expected in this clinical scenario and is generally associated with lower risk for seizure* (Figure 6.7).

2. **Medium risk**: A 55-year-old man presents after a focal-to-bilateral tonic clonic seizure, found to have large right MCA stroke. EEG showing frequent runs of blunted LPDs in the right parietal region at 0.5–1 Hz with some superimposed fast activity. The patient is encephalopathic with left hemiparesis. There is no response to a challenge with intravenous lorazepam. *This pattern warrants antiseizure medication, but it does not necessarily require aggressive treatment (e.g., suppression) given that the underlying structural lesion explains his ongoing neurological deficits* (Figure 6.8).

3. **High risk**: A 60-year-old woman with metastatic ovarian cancer who presents after a convulsive seizure and persistent encephalopathy, found to have metastatic disease in the brain. Continuous EEG shows continuous UiPDs fluctuating between 1 and 2 Hz. A challenge with intravenous lorazepam temporarily clears up the UiPD pattern, but there is no discernable improvement in clinical status. This pattern lies on the, IIC presents "possible" electroclinical status epilepticus, and escalation of treatment depends on the specific factors of the case. *Risks of escalating treatment must be carefully weighed against the potential benefit of improving the EEG pattern (which may be either ictal or interictal at this point)* (Figure 6.9).

4. **Highest risk/seizure**: A 35-year-old woman presents with encephalopathy and periods of unresponsiveness. Her EEG shows abundant generalized sharp-slow wave activity (GSW) at 1.5 Hz, which does not meet formal criteria for status epilepticus in and of itself. After a challenge of intravenous lorazepam 4 mg, the patient becomes more lucid and the GSW pattern dissipates, giving way to a normal EEG background. *This clinical scenario is considered electroclinical status epilepticus (ECSE), regardless of the specifics of the EEG pattern* (Figure 6.10).

Chapter 10 covers the topic of the treatment of RPPs lying on the IIC in greater depth.

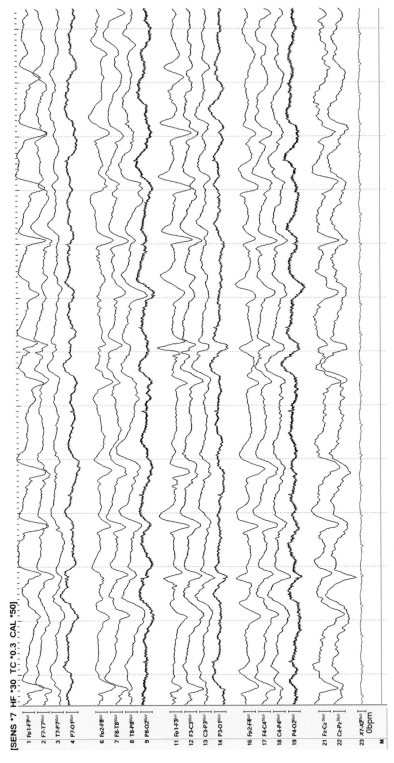

Figure 6.7 Low risk: periodic triphasic waves at 1 Hz.

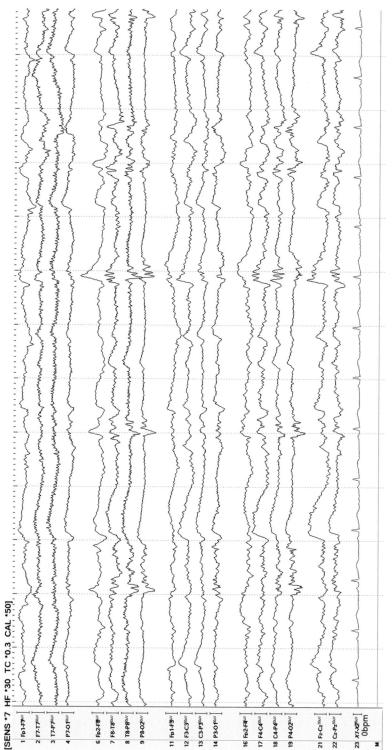

Figure 6.8 Medium risk: LPD+F (right posterior quadrant) at 0.5–1 Hz or less; meets criteria for IIC given the "+F" modifier.

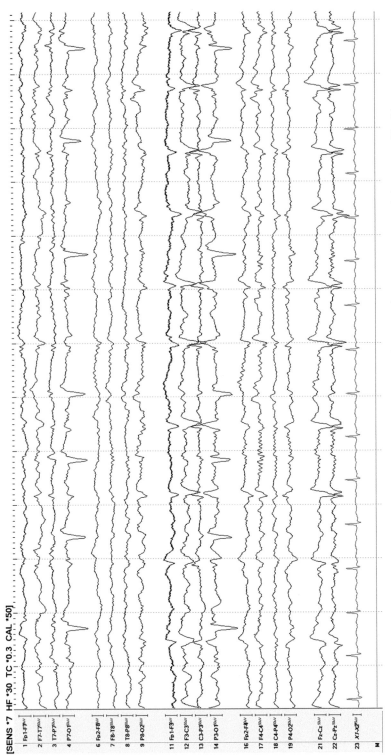

[SENS *7   HF *30   TC *0.3   CAL *50]

1 Fp1-F7⁽ᴬⱽ⁾
2 F7-T7⁽ᴬⱽ⁾
3 T7-P7⁽ᴬⱽ⁾
4 P7-O1⁽ᴬⱽ⁾

6 Fp2-F8⁽ᴬⱽ⁾
7 F8-T8⁽ᴬⱽ⁾
8 T8-P8⁽ᴬⱽ⁾
9 P8-O2⁽ᴬⱽ⁾

11 Fp1-F3⁽ᴬⱽ⁾
12 F3-C3⁽ᴬⱽ⁾
13 C3-P3⁽ᴬⱽ⁾
14 P3-O1⁽ᴬⱽ⁾

16 Fp2-F4⁽ᴬⱽ⁾
17 F4-C4⁽ᴬⱽ⁾
18 C4-P4⁽ᴬⱽ⁾
19 P4-O2⁽ᴬⱽ⁾

21 Fz-Cz⁽ᴬⱽ⁾
22 Cz-Pz⁽ᴬⱽ⁾
23 X1-X2⁽ᴬⱽ⁾

Figure 6.9 High risk: UIPDs at 1–1.5 Hz. Lies on the IIC, possible ECSE given only electrographic improvement with lorazepam IV, without clinical improvement.

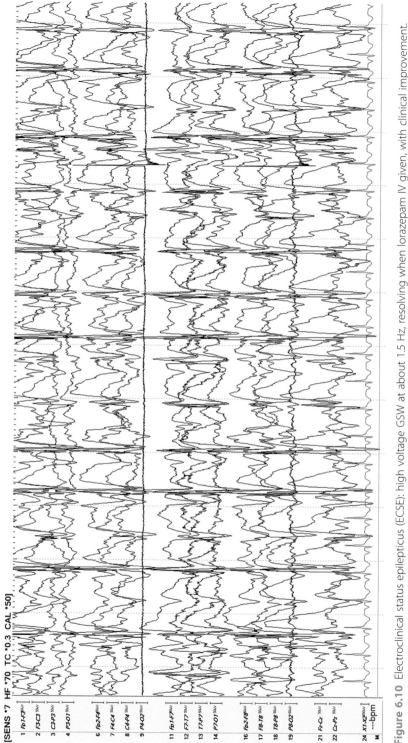

[SENS *7 HF *70 TC *0.3 CAL *50]

1 Fp1-F3 50µV
2 F3-C3 50µV
3 C3-P3 50µV
4 P3-O1 50µV

6 Fp2-F4 50µV
7 F4-C4 50µV
8 C4-P4 50µV
9 P4-O2 50µV

11 Fp1-F7 50µV
12 F7-T7 50µV
13 T7-P7 50µV
14 P7-O1 50µV

16 Fp2-F8 50µV
17 F8-T8 50µV
18 T8-P8 50µV
19 P8-O2 50µV

21 Fz-Cz 50µV
22 Cz-Pz 50µV

24 X1-X2 50µV
M ---bpm

Figure 6.10 Electroclinical status epilepticus (ECSE): high voltage GSW at about 1.5 Hz, resolving when lorazepam IV given, with clinical improvement.

References

1. Hirsch LJ, Fong MWK, Leitinger M, et al. American Clinical Neurophysiology Society's Standardized Critical Care EEG Terminology: 2021 version. *Journal of Clinical Neurophysiology.* 2021 Jan 1;38(1):1–29.

2. Trinka E, Cock H, Hesdorffer D, et al. A definition and classification of status epilepticus – Report of the ILAE Task Force on Classification of Status Epilepticus. *Epilepsia.* 2015 Oct;56(10):1515–23.

3. Gaspard N, Hirsch LJ, LaRoche SM, et al. Interrater agreement for Critical Care EEG Terminology. *Epilepsia.* 2014 Sep;55(9):1366–73.

4. Kaplan PW, Sutter R. Affair with triphasic waves – Their striking presence, mysterious significance, and cryptic origins: What are they? *Journal of Clinical Neurophysiology.* 2015 Oct;32(5):401–5.

5. Foreman B, Mahulikar A, Tadi P, et al. Generalized periodic discharges and 'triphasic waves': A blinded evaluation of inter-rater agreement and clinical significance. *Clinical Neurophysiology.* 2016 Feb;127(2):1073–80.

6. Chong DJ, Hirsch LJ. Which EEG patterns warrant treatment in the critically ill? Reviewing the evidence for treatment of periodic epileptiform discharges and related patterns. *Journal of Clinical Neurophysiology.* 2005 Apr;22(2):79–91.

7. Rubinos C, Reynolds AS, Claassen J. The ictal-interictal continuum: To treat or not to treat (and how)? *Neurocritical Care.* 2018 Aug;29(1):3–8.

8. Zafar SF, Subramaniam T, Osman G, et al. Electrographic seizures and ictal-interictal continuum (IIC) patterns in critically ill patients. *Epilepsy & Behavior.* 2020 May;106:107037.

7

Post–Cardiac Arrest EEG

- Continuous EEG monitoring following cardiac arrest
- Hypothermia protocols
- Continuous EEG use in neurological prognostication
- Standardized EEG interpretation can aid in predicting neurological outcomes

- Anoxic myoclonic status epilepticus
- Differentiating anoxic myoclonic status epilepticus from the Lance–Adams syndrome
- EEG in brain death protocols

Cardiac arrest often leads to diffuse hypoxic ischemic encephalopathy, a condition ranging from mild to neurologically devastating. Continuous EEG monitoring can aid in the prognostication of patients who have suffered cardiac arrest and suspected hypoxic ischemic brain injury (HIBI). In the proper clinical context, and when interpreted in a standardized way by an expert, specific EEG patterns can be benign or suggestive of a poor neurological prognosis.

Continuous EEG Monitoring preposition Cardiac Arrest

Continuous EEG monitoring is recommended following cardiac arrest [1]. In these patients CEEG is useful to:

- Aid in the detection of subclinical, nonconvulsive seizures that may not otherwise be detectable.
- Evaluate for EEG evidence of HIBI
- Provide supplementary evidence for neurological prognostication.

Hypothermia Protocols

Therapeutic hypothermia (TH) is employed after cardiac arrest to decrease the metabolic demands on the brain and reduce the odds or severity of

HIBI. During this critical time (especially rewarming following TH) patients may be at particular risk for seizures. Thus CEEG monitoring is recommended in patients following cardiac arrest until after the patient has been rewarmed [2].

Continuous EEG Use in Neurological Prognostication

EEG alone (continuous or otherwise) should not be used to estimate prognosis following cardiac arrest. Important considerations in making this estimation are:

- Clinical neurological exam
- Neuroimaging (e.g., MRI) and other modalities.
- Clinical history and comorbidities.

However, the EEG can supplement these to aid in prognostication. A number of EEG patterns may be seen after cardiac arrest (see Chapters 3, 5, and 6), however there are specific features outlined in the next section that may have particular implications.

Standardized EEG Interpretation Can Aid in Predicting Neurological Outcomes

The following EEG features correlate with poor neurological outcomes following cardiac arrest:

- **Burst suppression** (Figure 7.1). When at least 50% of the EEG record is suppressed ($<10\ \mu V$), this meets criteria for burst suppression, a deeper level of discontinuity. Some unique features of burst suppression that may be seen after cardiac arrest include:
  - ○ **Identical bursts.** Bursts appear stereotyped, and are particularly associated with poor neurological outcomes after cardiac arrest [3].
- **Generalized voltage suppression** (Figure 7.2): most or all EEG activity is suppressed ($<10\ \mu V$). Of note, a suppressed background on EEG does not necessarily equate to electrocerebral inactivity (ECI). ECI can only be determine using the specific brain death EEG protocol, which uses double distance electrodes and other specific recording parameters (see Chapter 15).
- **Lack of EEG reactivity** (Figure 7.3). When there is no discernable change in EEG frequency or pattern following escalating noxious stimulation (see Chapter 3), the EEG is considered to be unreactive, or lacks EEG-R.
- **"Malignant" rhythmic or periodic pattern (RPP)** (Figure 7.4). When an RPP is seen after cardiac arrest and consists of abundant periodic discharges (PDs), spike-wave (SW), or meets criteria for frank seizure, it is considered "malignant." Importantly, a recent randomized controlled trial concluded that suppressing these RPPs for 48 hours in comatose survivors of cardiac

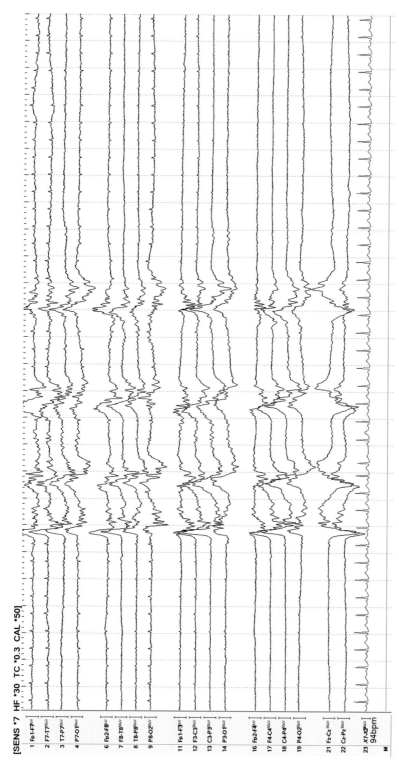

[SENS *7   HF *30   TC *0.3   CAL *50]

1 Fp1-F7
2 F7-T7
3 T7-P7
4 P7-O1

6 Fp2-F8
7 F8-T8
8 T8-P8
9 P8-O2

11 Fp1-F3
12 F3-C3
13 C3-P3
14 P3-O1

16 Fp2-F4
17 F4-C4
18 C4-P4
19 P4-O2

21 Fz-Cz
22 Cz-Pz

23 X1-X2
94bpm

M

Figure 7.1 Burst suppression with "identical bursts" following cardiac arrest; note the compressed time scale.

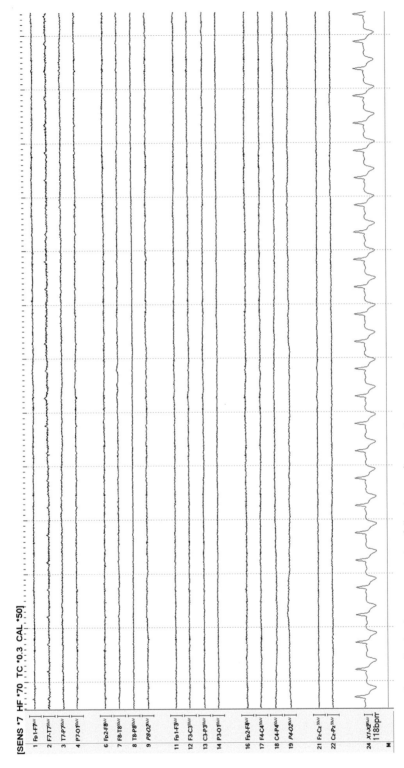

Figure 7.2 Generalized voltage suppression following cardiac arrest.

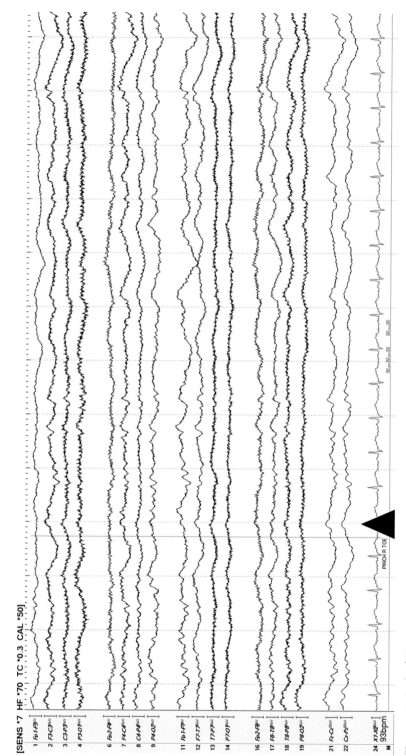

Figure 7.3 Lack of EEG reactivity (unreactive EEG) following cardiac arrest; reactivity testing with noxious stimulus is marked with a black arrow.

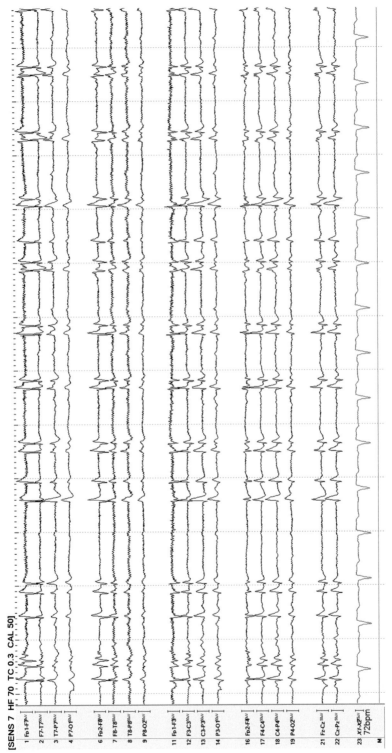

Figure 7.4 A "malignant" RPP following cardiac arrest. This pattern could be considered GPDs on a suppressed background, or burst suppression with highly epileptiform bursts.

arrest did not significantly change the incidence of poor neurological outcomes [4].

- **Seizures** (Figure 7.5). Frank seizures can be seen after cardiac arrest, ranging from small, focal, subclinical seizures to dramatic, generalized, myoclonic seizures.

A systematic review of EEG findings and outcomes following cardiac arrest found that no one EEG pattern is *invariably* associated with death or disability [5], but *status epilepticus, burst suppression,* and *suppressed background/ECI* correlated with poor neurological outcomes [5,6].

Another study found that two or more of these "malignant" EEG features occurring together following cardiac arrest predicted a higher likelihood of poor neurological prognosis [6].

Confounding factors such as TH, toxic metabolic abnormalities, and sedating medications should also be considered when estimating neurological prognosis.

Conversely, a continuous and reactive EEG background without epileptiform discharges within 72 hours of the cardiac arrest event may be associated with favorable outcomes [7].

Anoxic Myoclonic Status Epilepticus

Anoxic myoclonic status epilepticus (AMSE) is a particularly notorious electroclinical entity, representing a fulminant form of HIBI. It meets clinical criteria for status epilepticus and is characterized by sustained or recurrent myoclonic jerking (irregular or regular) and sometimes discrete myoclonic seizures [8]. The abnormal movements arise due to diffuse cortical injury, and on EEG there is abnormal epileptiform activity underlying the jerking movements, often in the form of an RPP (Figure 7.6). This condition is differentiated from subcortically generated myoclonus by the clear underlying EEG correlate. This pattern typically portends a poor neurological prognosis despite aggressive treatments [9].

Differentiating Anoxic Myoclonic Status Epilepticus from Lance–Adams Syndrome

While clinical diagnosis is beyond the scope of this book, it bears mentioning that it is critically important to differentiate AMSE from what is known as Lance–Adams syndrome [10], the latter being a more delayed form of post–cardiac arrest myoclonus. Patients with Lance–Adams syndrome can recover from cardiac arrest with varying degrees of neurological impairment. Consultation with a neurologist is recommended in these situations.

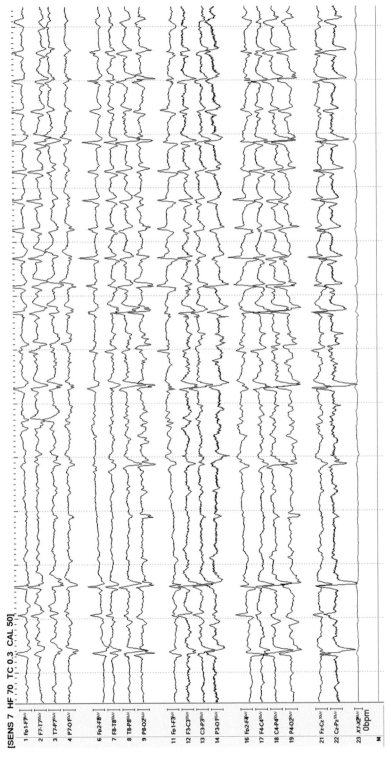

[SENS 7 HF 70 TC 0.3 CAL 50]

1 Fp1-F7$^{50\mu V}$
2 F7-T7$^{50\mu V}$
3 T7-P7$^{50\mu V}$
4 P7-O1$^{50\mu V}$

6 Fp2-F8$^{50\mu V}$
7 F8-T8$^{50\mu V}$
8 T8-P8$^{50\mu V}$
9 P8-O2$^{50\mu V}$

11 Fp1-F3$^{50\mu V}$
12 F3-C3$^{50\mu V}$
13 C3-P3$^{50\mu V}$
14 P3-O1$^{50\mu V}$

16 Fp2-F4$^{50\mu V}$
17 F4-C4$^{50\mu V}$
18 C4-P4$^{50\mu V}$
19 P4-O2$^{50\mu V}$

21 Fz-Cz$^{50\mu V}$
22 Cz-Pz$^{50\mu V}$

23 X1-X2$^{50\mu V}$
0bpm

M

Figure 7.5 Beginning of a seizure occurring after cardiac arrest.

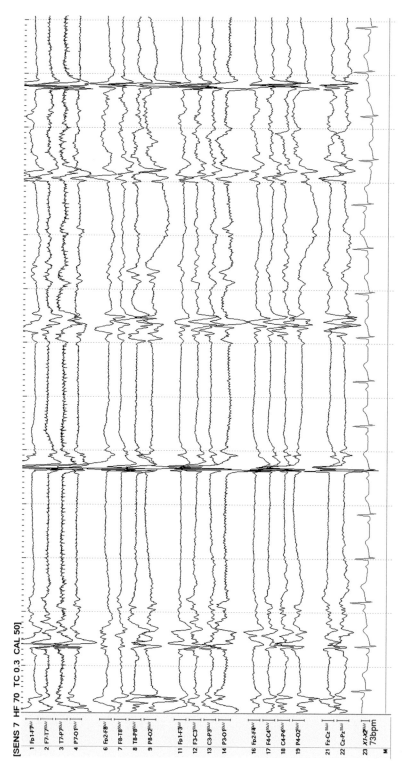

[SENS 7 HF 70 TC 0.3 CAL 50]

1 Fp1-F7[AV]
2 F7-T7[AV]
3 T7-P7[AV]
4 P7-O1[AV]

6 Fp2-F8[AV]
7 F8-T8[AV]
8 T8-P8[AV]
9 P8-O2[AV]

11 Fp1-F3[AV]
12 F3-C3[AV]
13 C3-P3[AV]
14 P3-O1[AV]

16 Fp2-F4[AV]
17 F4-C4[AV]
18 C4-P4[AV]
19 P4-O2[AV]

21 Fz-Cz[AV]
22 Cz-Pz[AV]

23 X1-X2[AV]
73bpm

Figure 7.6 EEG of anoxic myoclonic status epilepticus; in this case, movements are subtle and not creating significant artifact.

EEG in Brain Death Protocols

While EEG alone should not be used to determine brain death, it may be used as a supplementary tool to aid with determination of brain death. In this situation, the EEG should be performed using the specifications recommended by the American Clinical Neurophysiology Society [11]. This protocol uses double distance electrodes and higher sensitivity, and all waveforms must be explained if not attributed to cerebral activity.

A minimum of 30 minutes must be recorded in these cases. See Chapter 15 cases for additional information on this topic.

References

1. Herman ST, Abend NS, Bleck TP, et al. Consensus statement on continuous EEG in critically ill adults and children, Part I: Indications. *Journal of Clinical Neurophysiology*. 2015 Apr;32(2):87–95.
2. Sandroni C, Natalini D, Nolan JP. Temperature control after cardiac arrest. *Critical Care*. 2022 Nov 24;26(1):361.
3. Hofmeijer J, Tjepkema-Cloostermans MC, van Putten MJ. Burst-suppression with identical bursts: A distinct EEG pattern with poor outcome in postanoxic coma. *Clinical Neurophysiology*. 2014 May;125(5):947–54.
4. Ruijter BJ, Keijzer HM, Tjepkema-Cloostermans MC, et al. Treating rhythmic and periodic EEG patterns in comatose survivors of cardiac arrest. *New England Journal of Medicine*. 2022 Feb 24;386(8):724–34.
5. Perera K, Khan S, Singh S, et al. EEG patterns and outcomes after hypoxic brain injury: A systematic review and meta-analysis. *Neurocritical Care*. 2022 Feb;36(1):292–301.
6. Sethi NK, Westhall E, Rossetti AO, et al. Standardized EEG interpretation accurately predicts prognosis after cardiac arrest. *Neurology*. 2016 Oct 11;87(15):1631.
7. Sandroni C, D'Arrigo S, Cacciola S, et al. Prediction of good neurological outcome in comatose survivors of cardiac arrest: A systematic review. *Intensive Care Medicine*. 2022 Apr;48(4):389–413.
8. Bauer G, Unterberger I. Anoxic myoclonic status epilepticus. In Drislane FW, Kaplan PW (Eds.). *Status Epilepticus: A Clinical Perspective*. Second Edition. Springer Science+Business Media LLC, 2018.
9. Rossetti AO. Should postanoxic status epilepticus be treated aggressively? – No! *Journal of Clinical Neurophysiology*. 2015 Dec;32(6):447–8.
10. Freund B, Kaplan PW. Differentiating Lance-Adams syndrome from other forms of postanoxic myoclonus. *Annals of Neurology*. 2016 Dec;80(6):956.
11. Stecker MM, Sabau D, Sullivan L, et al. American Clinical Neurophysiology Society Guideline 6: Minimum Technical Standards for EEG Recording in Suspected Cerebral Death. *Journal of Clinical Neurophysiology*. 2016 Aug;33(4):324–7.

Quantitative EEG (EEG Trend Analysis)

- Efficiency of interpretation
- Amplitude integrated EEG (AIE)
- FFT spectrogram (FFTS)
- Rhythmicity spectrogram (RS)

- Asymmetry indices
- Seizure detectors
- Other trends
- Limitations

As the use of continuous EEG monitoring increases, electroencephalographers are reading more and more studies, which is time-consuming. Assuming a page length of 15 seconds and a reading speed of 5–10 pages per second (variable by reader), and assuming the reader reviewed every page of the study (our recommendation), a 24-hour continuous EEG study will take at the very least 10–20 minutes to review. Quantitative EEG (QEEG) aids in the rapid screening and even interpretation of EEG at a much faster speed, sometimes just at a glance.

Additionally, while we encourage non-neurologists and non-electroencephalographers to begin to take an active role in EEG reading, formal interpretation requires extensive training to properly interpret waveforms. Quantitative EEG trends simplifies many aspects of EEG reading and makes the process much more accessible to other types of providers.

Certain specific applications of QEEG have been determined. Common roles of QEEG in the ICU include the following [1,2]:

- Seizure detection
- Identifying and tracking the depth of burst suppression
- Detecting delayed cerebral ischemia (DCI) following subarachnoid hemorrhage (SAH)
- Post–cardiac arrest prognostication.

Key Principles
- QEEG is complementary to raw EEG, but **cannot** replace it.
- Always start with a review of the raw EEG to establish a baseline.

- Sudden changes in QEEG trends can be due to:
  - Seizure
  - State changes
  - Artifact
- Slow change in QEEG trends can be due to:
  - State changes
  - Rhythmic and periodic patterns (RPPs) and ictal-interictal continuum (IIC) patterns
  - Delayed cerebral ischemic (DCI) patterns.
- Short duration, low amplitude, low frequency, and slowly evolving seizures are difficult to detect on QEEG.

Efficiency of Interpretation

QEEG can be processed such that a time period ranging from minutes to 24 hours is visible on the monitor all at once, thus allowing the reader to view large swaths of time. This allows easy determination of changes and progression over time periods of these lengths. *Importantly, subtle details can be easily lost as the length of time increases.*

Shorter time windows are more useful for viewing seizures. Longer time windows are often more useful for viewing changes in background continuity, asymmetry, or the proportion of the record dominated by electrographic status epilepticus (ESE) and RPPs.

In general, the raw EEG signal is broken down into discrete numerical variables as follows:

- **Power** or **amplitude**: overall signal strength detected in the region of interest
- **Frequency**: speed of the signal or size of the wave as determined by the fast Fourier transformation (FFT)
- **Localization**: QEEG can process an entire hemisphere together for broad asymmetry analyses, or can focus on individual regions or EEG channels
- **Rhythmicity**: the temporal consistency of the EEG waves. Generalized rhythmic delta activity (GRDA) will be detected as rhythmic whereas arrhythmic polymorphic delta slowing will not be detected.

In QEEG, the raw EEG is processed by the variables above (sometimes after processing to remove the influence of artifacts), and plotted in various plots or spectral arrays to large periods of time at once. The different types of arrays generated are considered *complementary*, and one is not inherently better than the others. In general, the sum total of all of these methods is far more powerful than any of the individual processing methods in isolation [1].

However, given its lack of ability to differentiate the nuances of waveform morphology, QEEG analysis cannot substitute for interpretation of the raw EEG tracings.

Here, we will review the most common and useful QEEG trends you are likely to encounter.

Amplitude Integrated EEG

Description

Amplitude integrated EEG (AIE) is one of the simplest forms of quantitative EEG processing. It focuses on overall power of the signals, which is expressed in microvolts (μV). It plots minimal and maximal amplitude (voltage) within a given frequency range.

Applications

AIE differentiates differences in overall signal power between both hemispheres and can be programmed to look specifically at different locations. This can be useful for determining hemisphere asymmetry (focal slowing, focal voltage attenuation). It can also be helpful in looking at continuity versus discontinuity, given the stark contrast between periods of suppression and periods of cerebral activity.

AIE is perhaps best used for **seizure detection**. Abrupt increases in amplitude due to seizures can be detected as a dome shaped curve; a broken dome shaped curve usually arises from artifact.

Examples of AIE can be found in the "E" panels of Figures 8.1–8.4.

FFT Spectrogram

Description

The fast Fourier transformation spectrogram (FFTS) (power spectral array) is the most colorful of the QEEG trends and contains more information than AIE. The most important differentiating feature is the inclusion of frequency data, which is determined by the FFT technique.

The FFTS is a three-axis array with time on the x-axis, frequency on the y-axis, and power on the z-axis, determined by color intensity. The individual color paradigm is variable (see legend when available), but most commonly dark black/blue colors represent low power, and hotter colors (e.g., red/white) represent higher power in a given frequency range. Of note, individuals with color blindness may need the color scheme adjusted.

Applications

Over short time periods, FFTS allows visualization of frequency changes (including the evolution in seizures) and is one of many ways in which seizures can be more easily visualized. FFTS is useful in seeing normal sleep cycling (slow wave sleep), state changes in encephalopathic patients, and seizures. FFTS alone is weaker in determining asymmetries given the lack of overlapping graphs on the most basic algorithms.

Examples of FFTS can be found in the "C" panels of Figures 8.1–8.4.

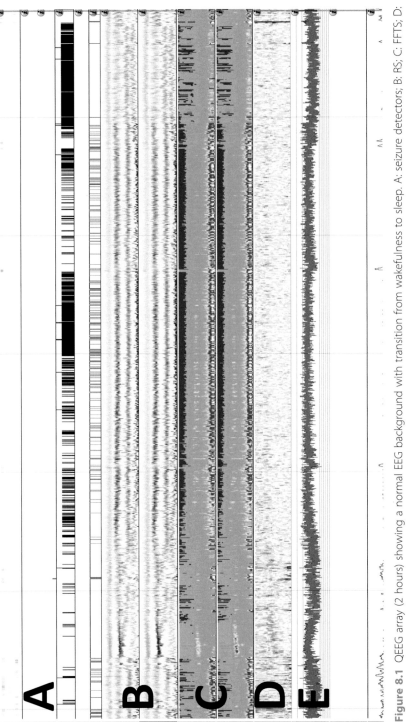

Figure 8.1 QEEG array (2 hours) showing a normal EEG background with transition from wakefulness to sleep. A: seizure detectors; B: RS; C: FFTS; D: asymmetry spectrogram; E: AIE.

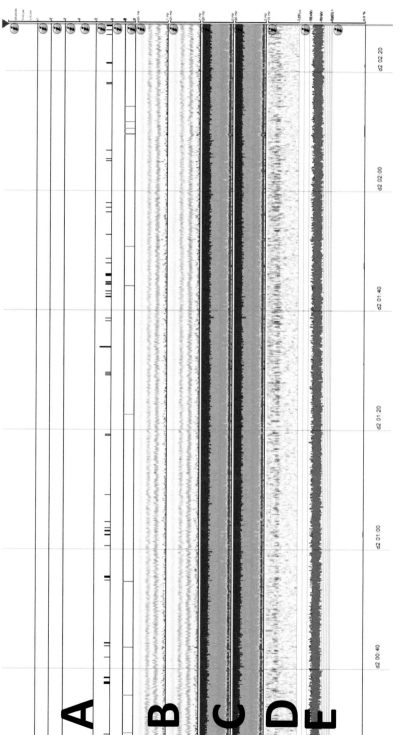

Figure 8.2 QEEG array (2 hours) showing a slow and unreactive background. A: seizure detectors; B: RS; C: FFTS; D: asymmetry spectrogram; E: AIE.

Rhythmicity Spectrogram

Description

Rhythmicity spectrogram (RS) is similar to the power spectral assay (PSA) but, rather than focusing on the power of signals, the algorithms favor regular/rhythmic signals. In these arrays, the yellow/beige color represents the background and arrhythmic/polymorphic signals, and the darker colors represent higher voltage, more clearly rhythmic signals. Like the FFTS, frequency is denoted on the y-axis.

Applications

This spectrogram is useful for viewing many normal and abnormal rhythms ranging from the PDR in awake patients to GRDA and LRDA, LPDs and GPDs, and most importantly seizures.

As the frequency of the signal of RPPs like GPDs increases, the RS signal rises accordingly, allowing easy visualization of fluctuating or evolving frequencies of these potentially concerning patterns.

While the default type of RS separates signals broadly between the hemispheres, the individual focus of the RS can be resolved to the level of individual channels of the EEG, which can be quite sensitive for the detective of focal seizures when programmed appropriately.

Examples of RS can be found in the "B" panels of Figures 8.1–8.4.

Asymmetry Indices

Description

The asymmetry index takes many forms and can be based on either AIE or FFTS. The focus of asymmetry indices is to show the differences in either overall power or specific frequency range between the two hemispheres (by default) in a quantitative, visual way. However, the settings can be adjusted to focus on determining the asymmetry between specific areas of the brain, ranging from quadrants to specific channels.

In the AIE-based methods (older), deflection in one direction or the other from baseline indicated a difference in power between the hemispheres. The power between homologous electrodes (e.g., T7 vs. T8) is compared directly. Upward deflection implies more power on the right and downward deflection is left.

In the FFTS-based algorithms (newer), color is used to denote asymmetries. Preponderance in a given frequency range in the left hemisphere is blue, and in the right hemisphere it is red; the deeper the color, the stronger the asymmetry.

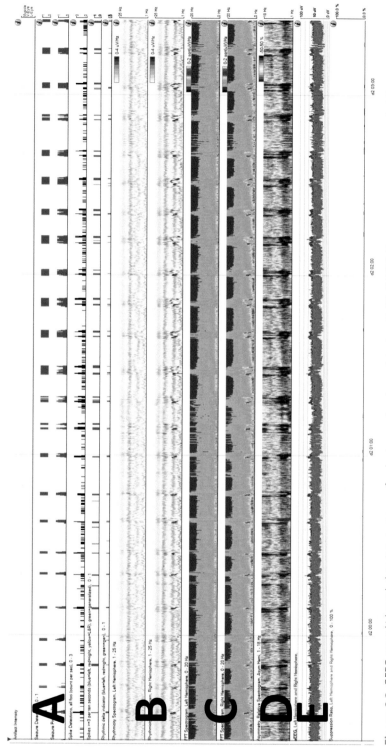

Figure 8.3 QEEG array (4 hours) showing numerous focal seizures. A: seizure detectors; B: RS; C: FFTS; D: asymmetry spectrogram; E: AIE.

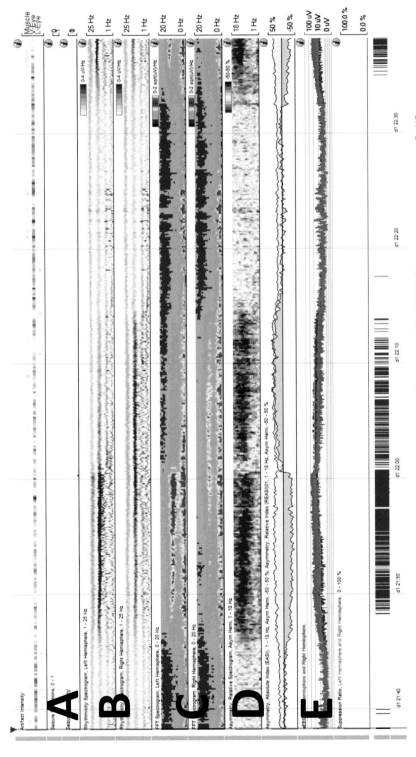

Figure 8.4 QEEG array (60 minutes) showing a focal seizure. A: seizure detectors; B: RS; C: FFTS; D: asymmetry spectrogram; E: AIE.

Applications

This spectrogram is useful for determining asymmetry that can be caused by focal slowing, focal voltage attenuation, breach effects, postictal findings, or focal seizures. This can be useful to detect in which hemisphere a seizure starts, and how it spreads.

Examples of asymmetry spectrograms can be found in the "D" panels of Figures 8.1–8.4.

Seizure Detectors

Any or all of the individual methods described can be used to detect seizures [3], though none of them is as useful as all of them together. Like in raw EEG, the detection of individual seizures is determined by discrete episodes (>10 seconds) of evolving rhythmic EEG signals, evolving in frequency (as seen on FFTS, RS), and topology (AI when programmed, but raw EEG will be more useful here aside from bilateral spread). Evolution in morphology is much better assessed by the raw EEG; this is an inherent weakness of QEEG.

Seizure, as determined by runs of GPDs or LPDs >2.5 Hz >10 seconds, can also be detected by the RS in many cases, though it is always necessary to verify the frequency and any *fluctuations* or *evolution* on the raw EEG. QEEG is not precise when dealing with IIC patterns.

Once a given seizure pattern has been confirmed in a given patient, it is generally much easier to know whether or not the detected pattern is a seizure.

Seizure detections made by automated algorithms always must be verified by review of the raw EEG, as various artifacts including suctioning, chest PT, chewing, and others can produce artifacts on the EEG that will be detected as seizures.

Examples of the "seizure detector" algorithm can be found in the "A" panels of Figures 8.1–8.4, though only Figure 8.3 shows positive detections.

While automated seizure detectors are often helpful, sometimes review of individual spectral arrays (or the raw EEG) can detect seizures that are missed. These are typically lower in voltage and more obscured by the background frequencies.

Concordance of multiple trends is most important when making an inference such as seizure detection. Many patients will have only one type of seizure pattern, so consistent patterns deserve close scrutiny.

In fact, specific detectors may be more useful to detect certain seizure subtypes [4]:

- **Asymmetry spectrogram:** highest sensitivity for detecting focal seizures
- **FFT spectrogram:** most sensitive for detecting secondarily generalized seizures
- **Seizure detection trend:** most sensitive for generalized onset seizures.

Other Trends
Additional QEEG trends not mentioned previously, but with specific clinical utility, include:

Burst Suppression Ratio
- Best used for determining the degree of suppression during periods of burst suppression.
- Plots the percentage of time the EEG is suppressed within a fixed time span.
- A flat line at the top represents a 100% suppressed background, and dips in the line indicate less suppression.
- Dips may be due to seizures (especially if dome shaped), but this is not the best QEEG trend marker for seizures.

Alpha–Delta Ratio
- Useful for delayed cerebral ischemia (DCI) in subarachnoid hemorrhage (SAH) [5].

Enveloped Trend (Peak Envelop)
- Good for detecting long and monotonous seizures; brief seizures can be missed.

Limitations and Caveats
Like raw EEG, QEEG is heavily affected by the presence of various artifacts that, when present and pronounced, can render the QEEG output useless in the worst cases.

Certain manufacturers have developed proprietary artifact reduction algorithms using individual component analysis to detect and subtract artifactual signals from the raw EEG tracing *prior* to doing the QEEG processing. Artifacts reduced include myogenic artifacts, blink artifacts, lateral eye movements, and some electrode-based artifacts. When an individual electrode is clearly not functioning properly, it is simply excluded from the processing altogether. This leads to much more reliable QEEG output, but unfortunately it is not foolproof.

When the QEEG does not look clean, review of the raw EEG is essential. Artifact reduction can be critical to the successful use of QEEG. Figures 8.5(a) and (b) show an example of a seizure on QEEG before and after the use of artifact reduction.

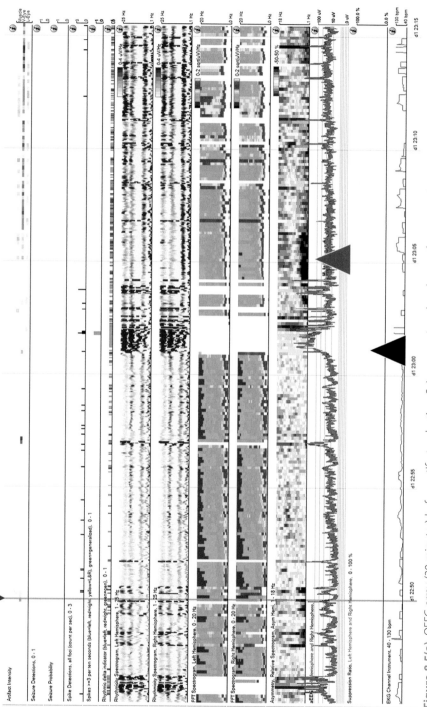

Figure 8.5(a) QEEG array (30 minutes) before artifact reduction. Seizure creating abundant artifact is noted with a black arrow; note the postictal right hemisphere slowing (red arrow).

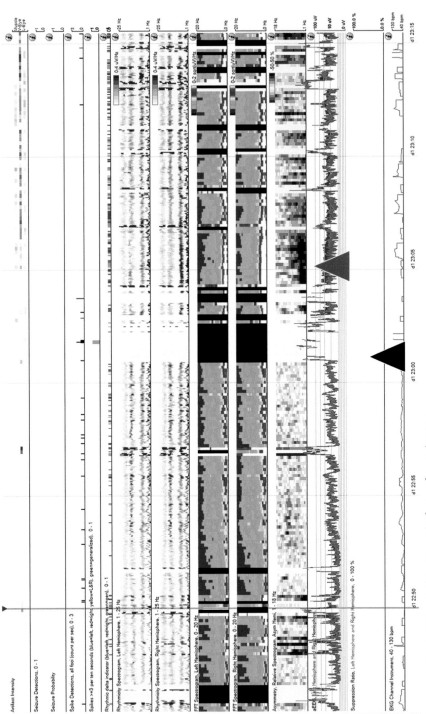

Artifact Intensity

Seizure Detections, 0 - 1

Seizure Probability

Spike Detections, all foci (count per sec), 0 - 3

Spikes >=3 per ten seconds (blue=left, red=right, yellow=L&R), green=generalized), 0 - 1

Rhythmic delta indicator (blue=left, red=right, green=gen), 0 - 1

Rhythmicity Spectrogram, Left Hemisphere, 1 - 25 Hz

Rhythmicity Spectrogram, Right Hemisphere, 1 - 25 Hz

FFT Spectrogram, Left Hemisphere, 0 - 20 Hz

FFT Spectrogram, Right Hemisphere, 0 - 20 Hz

Asymmetry, Relative Spectrogram, Asym Hemi, 1 - 18 Hz

aEEG Hemisphere and Right Hemisphere

Suppression Ratio, Left Hemisphere and Right Hemisphere, 0 - 100 %

EKG Channel Instrument, 40 -130 bpm

Figure 8.5(b) QEEG array (30 minutes) after artifact reduction.

References

1. Tong S, Thankor NV. *Quantitative EEG Analysis Methods and Clinical Applications.* Artech House, 2009.
2. Hwang J, Cho SM, Ritzl EK. Recent applications of quantitative electroencephalography in adult intensive care units: A comprehensive review. *Journal of Neurology.* 2022 Dec;269(12):6290–309.
3. Kaleem S, Swisher CB. Utility of quantitative EEG for seizure detection in adults. *Journal of Clinical Neurophysiology.* 2022 Mar 1;39(3):184–94.
4. Goenka A, Boro A, Yozawitz E. Comparative sensitivity of quantitative EEG (QEEG) spectrograms for detecting seizure subtypes. *Seizure.* 2018 Feb;55:70–5.
5. Baang HY, Chen HY, Herman AL, et al. The utility of quantitative EEG in detecting delayed cerebral ischemia after aneurysmal subarachnoid hemorrhage. *Journal of Clinical Neurophysiology.* 2022 Mar 1;39(3):207–15.

Case-Based Approach to Specific Conditions

Nonconvulsive Status Epilepticus (NCSE)

Learning Points
- Diagnosis of NCSE
- Types of NCSE

- Management of NCSE
- Refractory SE
- Absence SE

Case A 65-year-old woman with drug-resistant epilepsy presents to the ER with persistent confusion after multiple generalized tonic clonic seizures. Figure 9.1 shows a snapshot of her EEG.

How would you describe the EEG findings?
> *The EEG (Figure 9.1) shows continuous generalized spike-wave (GSW) discharges that occur at a frequency of about 3–4 Hz.*

What is your interpretation?
> *Continuous epileptic discharges occurring at a frequency >2.5 Hz are electrographically consistent with a diagnosis of electrographic status epilepticus (ESE) and clinically consistent with NCSE.*
>
> *Further, since these discharges have a "generalized" distribution (i.e., equally over both hemispheres), they are indicative of **generalized** NCSE.*

The next section describes how to make a diagnosis of NCSE.

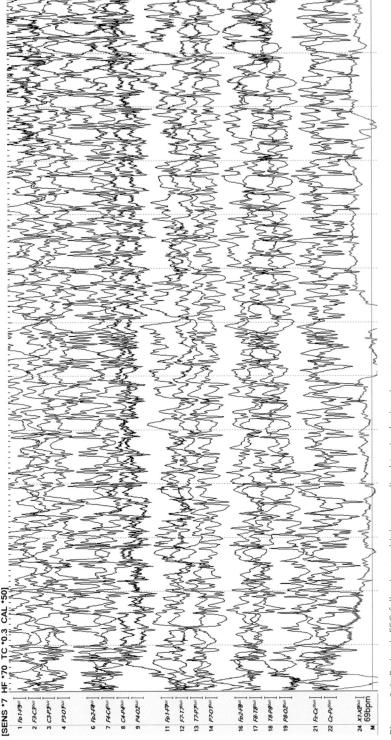

[SENS *7 HF *70 TC *0.3 CAL *50]

1 Fp1-F3ᴺⱽ
2 F3-C3ᴺⱽ
3 C3-P3ᴺⱽ
4 P3-O1ᴺⱽ

6 Fp2-F4ᴺⱽ
7 F4-C4ᴺⱽ
8 C4-P4ᴺⱽ
9 P4-O2ᴺⱽ

11 Fp1-F7ᴺⱽ
12 F7-T7ᴺⱽ
13 T7-P7ᴺⱽ
14 P7-O1ᴺⱽ

16 Fp2-F8ᴺⱽ
17 F8-T8ᴺⱽ
18 T8-P8ᴺⱽ
19 P8-O2ᴺⱽ

21 Fz-Cz³⁰ᵘⱽ
22 Cz-Pz³⁰ᵘⱽ

24 X1-X2ᴺⱽ
M   69bpm

Figure 9.1 Patient's EEG following multiple generalized tonic clonic seizures.

Diagnosis of NCSE

Continuous epileptiform discharges (spikes, sharp waves, polyspikes, spike-wave) occurring at a frequency ≥ 2.5 **Hz** confirm the diagnosis of NCSE.

However, if epileptic discharges occur at a frequency ≤ 2.5 **Hz,** or if rhythmic delta activity (RDA) is present, then making a diagnosis of NCSE requires at least one of the following secondary criteria:

(a) Subtle clinical phenomena (e.g., facial twitching), or
(b) Spatiotemporal evolution of epileptic activity, or
(c) Electrographic **and** clinical improvement after trial of an intravenous antiseizure medication (IV-ASM).

This definition uses the "Salzburg criteria" for diagnosing NCSE. Let's now apply it using a few more cases [1].

Case A 58-year-old man with multiple sclerosis presents with prolonged episodes of aphasia and confusion. Figure 9.2(a) shows a snapshot of his EEG.

How would you describe the EEG findings?
The EEG (Figure 9.2(a)) shows lateralized periodic discharges (LPDs) from the left posterior quadrant that occur at about 0.5–1 Hz.

What is your interpretation?
Although the above discharges occur at a frequency <2.5 Hz, they are consistent with a diagnosis of NCSE given they are associated with a concurrent associated clinical phenomenon – aphasia (secondary criterion (a) to make a diagnosis of NCSE in patients whose epileptic discharges occur at <2.5 Hz).

*Further, since these discharges have a "focal" distribution (i.e., limited to a single hemisphere), they are indicative of **focal** NCSE.*

Of note, during some aphasic episodes, the EEG pattern observed can be as shown in Figure 9.2(b).
How would you describe the EEG findings?
The EEG (Figure 9.2(b)) shows sharply contoured left temporal lateralized rhythmic delta activity (LRDA).

What is your interpretation?
Although the RDA appears "less sharp," its practical implication is the same as epileptic discharges at <2.5 Hz (i.e., the diagnosis of NCSE again requires at least one secondary criterion – in this case, aphasia).

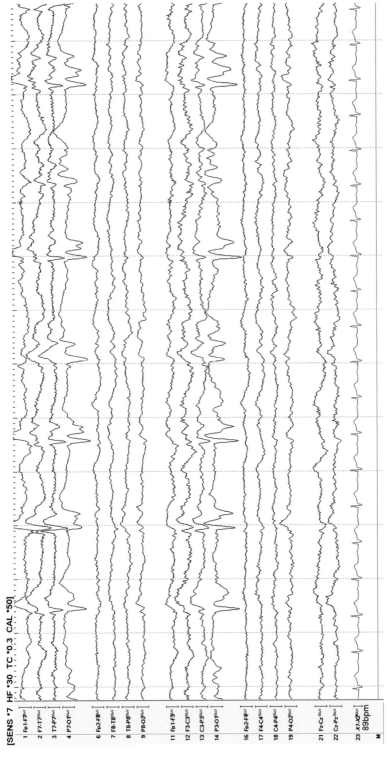

[SENS *7   HF *30   TC *0.3   CAL *50]

1 Fp1-F7^{50uV}
2 F7-T7^{50uV}
3 T7-P7^{50uV}
4 P7-O1^{50uV}

6 Fp2-F8^{50uV}
7 F8-T8^{50uV}
8 T8-P8^{50uV}
9 P8-O2^{50uV}

11 Fp1-F3^{50uV}
12 F3-C3^{50uV}
13 C3-P3^{50uV}
14 P3-O1^{50uV}

16 Fp2-F4^{50uV}
17 F4-C4^{50uV}
18 C4-P4^{50uV}
19 P4-O2^{50uV}

21 Fz-Cz^{50uV}
22 Cz-Pz^{50uV}

23 X1-X2^{50uV}
89bpm

Figure 9.2(a) Patient's EEG after prolonged episodes of aphasia and confusion.

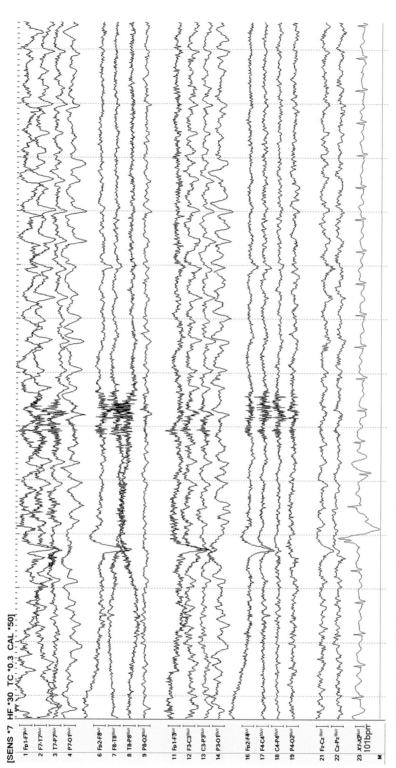

[SENS *7 HF *30 TC *0.3 CAL *50]

1 Fp1-F7
2 F7-T7
3 T7-P7
4 P7-O1

6 Fp2-F8
7 F8-T8
8 T8-P8
9 P8-O2

11 Fp1-F3
12 F3-C3
13 C3-P3
14 P3-O1

16 Fp2-F4
17 F4-C4
18 C4-P4
19 P4-O2

21 Fz-Cz
22 Cz-Pz

23 X1-X2
101bpm

Figure 9.2(b) Patient's EEG during an aphasic episode.

Case A 64-year-old lady with post-stroke epilepsy presents with sudden-onset confusion and worsening right hemiparesis. Figure 9.3 shows a snapshot of her EEG.

How would you describe the EEG findings?

The far left (Figure 9.3) shows 2 Hz LPDs (left temporal), which in time "evolve" in frequency and morphology to 5 Hz sharply contoured rhythmic theta activity (middle).

Further, this activity begins to spread outside the region of its onset (left temporal) into the left paracentral region (far right).

What is your interpretation?

*This is an **evolving pattern** as it shows sequential changes in frequency, morphology (shape), and location (space).*

Spatiotemporal evolution is another secondary criterion for a diagnosis of NCSE (if epileptic discharges ≤2.5 Hz or RDA). It is described further in Chapter 10, Management of the Ictal-Interictal Continuum.

Case A 64-year-old man with a history of COPD presents with acute onset encephalopathy. Figure 9.4(a) shows a snapshot of his initial EEG.

Figure 9.4(b) shows a snapshot of his EEG a few minutes after the administration of 2 mg IV lorazepam. The patient's mental status also transiently improves after receiving the IV-ASM.

How would you describe the EEG findings?

Initially, the EEG (Figure 9.4(a)) shows lateralized (focal) RDA with superimposed spikes (LRDA+S) over the right hemisphere spreading to the central regions.

After the administration of IV lorazepam (Figure 9.4(b)), LRDA+S resolves and there is diffuse beta activity and gradual restoration of background activity, accompanied by an appreciable clinical improvement as noted at the bedside.

What is your interpretation?

*Electrographic **and** clinical improvement following the administration of an IV-ASM is another secondary criterion for a diagnosis of NCSE (for epileptiform discharges ≤2.5 Hz or RDA).*

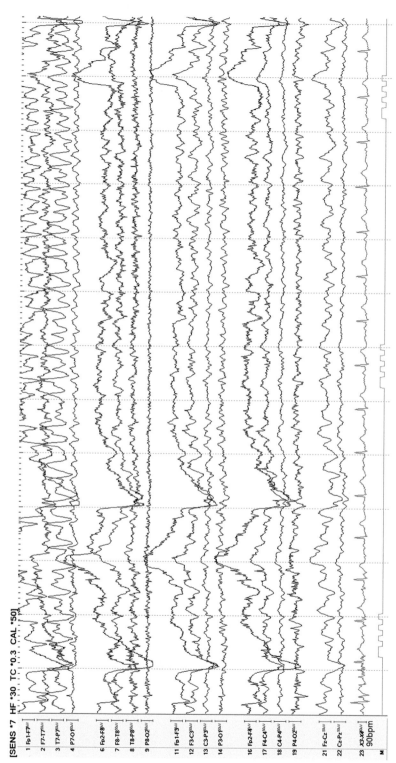

Figure 9.3 Patient's EEG after sudden-onset confusion and worsening right hemiparesis.

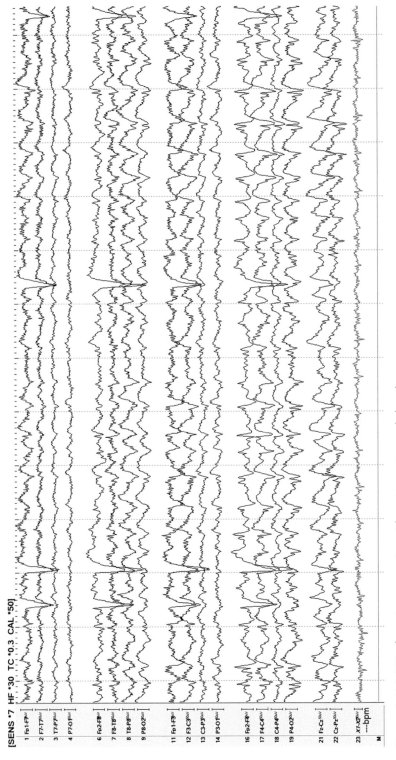

Figure 9.4(a) EEG of a patient presenting with acute onset encephalopathy.

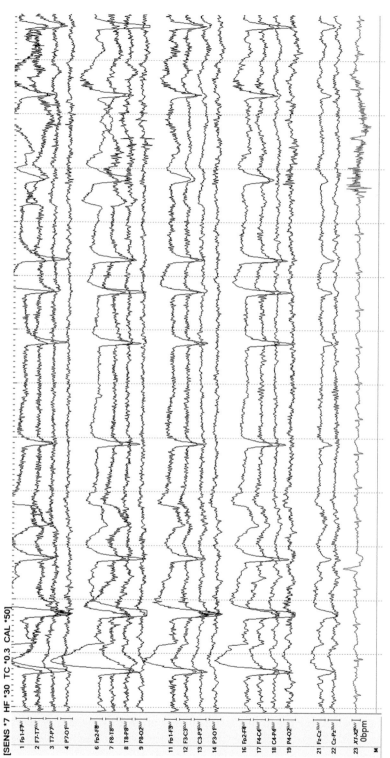

Figure 9.4(b) Patient's EEG after 2 mg IV lorazepam.

Clinical improvement can be determined at the bedside based on an improvement in mental status examination.

Usually, improvement will occur within a few minutes of receiving an IV-ASM (e.g., benzodiazepine), though it may lag by several hours especially if non-benzodiazepine IV-ASMs are used.

Electrographic improvement refers to a reduction in epileptic discharges or RDA as well as a gradual restoration of (previously absent) background activities such as the emergence of posterior dominant rhythm [2,3].

Of note, suppression of the record after the administration of a sedative by itself does not constitute "electrographic improvement."

Types of NCSE

As described earlier, NCSE may be classified based on semiology and EEG findings as focal or generalized.

Most "generalized" NCSE occurs secondary to focal onset with bilateral spread (secondary generalization). Less common primary generalized forms include absence SE.

Generalized NCSE, depending on its etiology, is associated with various degrees of severity of **impaired awareness**, including delirium and coma, or it may also be seen in those who are comatose due to another etiology such as anoxic or traumatic brain injury.

Focal NCSE typically occurs secondary to focal brain lesions. It may be suspected in those with unexplained/worsening **focal neurological deficits** with or without impaired awareness. Common manifestations include continuous aphasia, or sensory, visual, olfactory, emotional/psychic, or auditory aura depending on the region of cortical involvement (aura continua).

For example, word-finding difficulty (aphasia) typically occurs with left hemispheric (dominant lobe), and hemineglect with right hemispheric (non-dominant lobe) involvement. Frontal lobe involvement may manifest as contralateral gaze deviation, subtle motor activity, or hemiparesis. Sensory symptoms may suggest parietal lobe involvement; olfactory, emotional/psychic, or auditory symptoms may be associated with the temporal lobes; and visual symptoms may indicate occipital involvement.

NCSE may be further classified based on etiology (known/cryptogenic), EEG correlates, and age of onset [4].

Management of NCSE

Parenterally (usually IV) administered benzodiazepine (e.g., lorazepam 4 mg IV push, repeated every 5 minutes to a maximum of 0.1 mg/kg) along with an assessment and management of airway, breathing, and circulation, as well as a correction of potential metabolic abnormalities (e.g., hypoglycemia or thiamine deficiency), constitute the immediate first steps in the treatment of generalized SE. Intranasal, buccal, rectal, or intramuscular benzodiazepine alternatives should be considered in those lacking immediate IV access.

Table 9.1 Suggested load of IV-ASMs

Antiseizure medication*	Loading dose	Comments
Fosphenytoin (FOS)	20 mg PE/kg	Max 150 mg PE/min
Phenytoin (PHT)	20 mg/kg (may follow with an additional 10 mg/kg if no effect)	Max 50 mg/min (ECG/BP monitoring)
Valproate (VPA)	40 mg/kg	Max 6 mg/kg/min
Levetiracetam (LEV)	60 mg/kg (not exceeding 4.5 g)	Max 100 mg/min
Brivaracetam (BRV)	100 mg	Over 15 min
Lacosamide (LCM)	200–400 mg	Over 30 min (pre- and post-infusion ECG monitor for PR interval prolongation)
Phenobarbital (PB)	20 mg/kg	Max 50–75 mg/min

*Not all medications are FDA-approved for this purpose. PE, phenytoin equivalent.

If seizures persist, promptly follow with a loading dose of one or a combination of IV-ASMs ("second-line agents," see Table 9.1). These include phenytoin (or fosphenytoin), sodium valproate, levetiracetam, lacosamide, and/or phenobarbital. Brivaracetam may be an alternative to levetiracetam in those with impaired renal function.

Generalized SE (including NCSE) is a neurological emergency that is best managed in an ICU accompanied with continuous EEG monitoring. However, the optimal management of focal NCSE is less well defined. Concurrent efforts should be made to evaluate and treat the underlying cause of SE along with its immediate medical management [5].

Case A 68-year-old man with prior epilepsy presents with SE. He fails to respond to lorazepam and subsequent IV loading doses of levetiracetam and fosphenytoin. He is intubated and sedated with midazolam and propofol. Figure 9.5(a) shows a snapshot of his EEG.

How will you describe the EEG findings?
   The EEG (Figure 9.5(a)) shows a low voltage burst-suppressed background with ~1 second bursts and long interburst intervals.

What is your interpretation?
   These findings suggest that this patient with refractory SE is now adequately "burst suppressed."

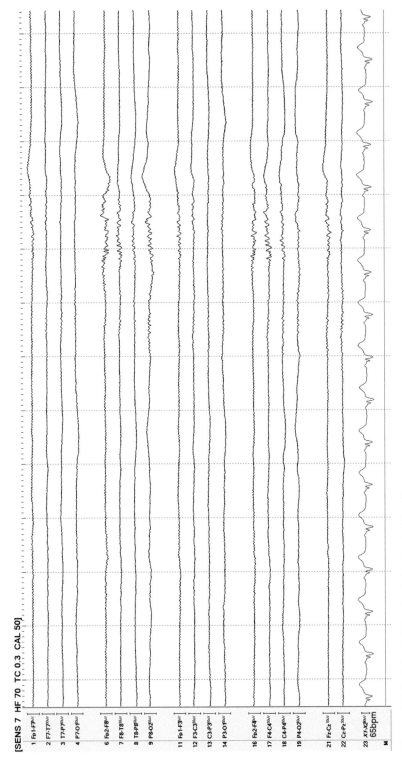

[SENS 7 HF 70 TC 0.3 CAL 50]

1 Fp1-F7^{50V}
2 F7-T7^{50uV}
3 T7-P7^{50uV}
4 P7-O1^{50uV}

6 Fp2-F8^{50uV}
7 F8-T8^{50uV}
8 T8-P8^{50uV}
9 P8-O2^{50uV}

11 Fp1-F3^{50uV}
12 F3-C3^{50uV}
13 C3-P3^{50uV}
14 P3-O1^{50uV}

16 Fp2-F4^{50uV}
17 F4-C4^{50uV}
18 C4-P4^{50uV}
19 P4-O2^{50uV}

21 Fz-Cz^{50uV}
22 Cz-Pz^{50uV}

23 X1-X2^{50uV}
65bpm

M

Figure 9.5(a) Patient's EEG after being treated for SE.

Table 9.2 Suggested loading and maintenance doses of IV anesthetics

Medication	Loading dose	Maintenance
Midazolam	0.2 mg/kg (max 2 mg/kg)	0.1–2 mg/kg/hour
Propofol	2 mg/kg (max 10 mg/kg)	1–10 mg/kg/hour
Pentobarbital	5 mg/kg (max 15 mg/kg)	1–10 mg/kg/hour

Refractory SE
- Failure of SE to terminate despite initial benzodiazepine and additional IV-ASMs is called refractory SE (RSE).
- About a third of all those with SE become refractory.
- A longer duration of SE (due to diagnostic delays, underdosing, or failure to treat underlying causes) may contribute to refractoriness.
- At this point, the patient should be intubated and placed on CEEG monitoring, preferably in an intensive care setting.
- IV infusion of midazolam or propofol is recommended.
- RSE is associated with a mortality of 30–60%. Those with known epilepsy may have a better prognosis [6,7].

How to Titrate to Burst Suppression
The infusion of IV anesthetics (e.g., midazolam, propofol or pentobarbital; see Table 9.2) should be titrated to achieve seizure termination or burst suppression. However, the optimal depth and duration of burst suppression is still unclear.

Common practice involves burst suppression titrated to 1–2 second bursts with ~10 second interburst intervals for an initial duration of 24 hours. However, ultrashort durations (<2 hours) have been successful (especially if clear seizure cessation is achieved) [8].

> **Case** After about 24 hours of burst suppression, a slow taper of IV anesthetics is attempted. Figure 9.5(b) shows a snapshot of the patient's EEG.
>
> How would you describe the EEG findings?
> *The EEG (Figure 9.5(b)) shows the emergence of abundant focal (left frontal) polyspike discharges within bursts with a reduction of burst suppression.*
>
> What is your interpretation?
> *Multiple epileptiform discharges within bursts are called highly epileptiform bursts (HEBs). These are associated with SE recurrence.*

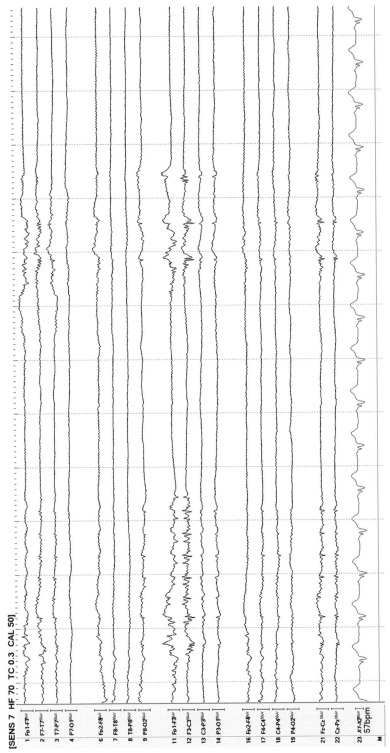

Figure 9.5(b) Patient's EEG after tapering IV anesthetics.

Super-Refractory SE (SRSE)

SE despite over 24 hours of anesthesia, or recurrence upon attempting to wean anesthetics, is called SRSE.

- Confirm the therapeutic levels of maintenance ASMs before attempting to wean IV anesthesia to reduce the risk of SE recurrence.

How to Recognize SRSE (Failure to Wean Anesthesia)

SRSE means the continuation or recurrence of SE despite adequate burst suppression. **Burst morphology** (not depth or duration of suppression) is a key determinant of seizure recurrence if anesthesia is tapered.

- Seizure recurrence is more likely when most bursts (>50%) contain embedded spikes/sharps, or if **highly epileptiform bursts** (HEBs; i.e., two or more spikes/sharps within each burst) occur.
- Conversely, the emergence of low-amplitude, polymorphic bursts without embedded discharges may indicate successful anesthetic withdrawal [9,10].

  Figure 9.5(c) shows a failure to taper IV anesthesia (SRSE) in this case.

How to Recognize SE Cessation (Stop, Stutter, or Slowly Fade Away)

Cessation of SE is marked by the termination of ictal activity and (often gradual) return of background activities, but not necessarily normal rhythms such as a reactive posterior dominant rhythm.

Usually, attenuation and slowing occur in the immediate postictal period followed by the restoration of baseline background activities.

Common EEG patterns of seizure cessation include:

- Abrupt halt (**stop**): ictal activity abruptly terminates followed by (>10 seconds of) nonictal activities such as background attenuation and slowing.
- Offset occurs with bursts (**stutter**): successive bursts of ictal activity, each interrupted by lengthening interburst intervals.
- Offset occurs with rhythmic/periodic patterns (**slowly fade away**): end manifests with nonictal PDs or RDA (<2.5 Hz, no clinical symptoms or EEG evolution).

After SE terminates, PDs or RDA may return to their preictal patterns or become slower, less sharp, and gradually fade away. Figure 9.6 shows a schematic representation of the above patterns.

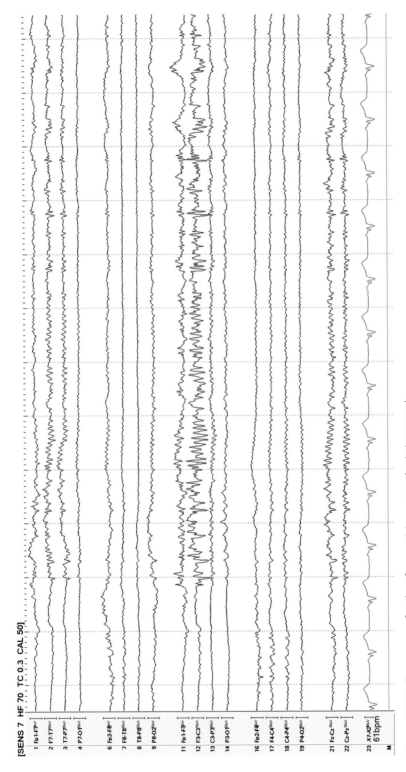

[SENS 7 HF 70 TC 0.3 CAL 50]

1 Fp1-F7⁽ᴿᴬᵁ⁾
2 F7-T7⁽ᴿᴬᵁ⁾
3 T7-P7⁽ᴿᴬᵁ⁾
4 P7-O1⁽ᴿᴬᵁ⁾

6 Fp2-F8⁽ᴿᴬᵁ⁾
7 F8-T8⁽ᴿᴬᵁ⁾
8 T8-P8⁽ᴿᴬᵁ⁾
9 P8-O2⁽ᴿᴬᵁ⁾

11 Fp1-F3⁽ᴿᴬᵁ⁾
12 F3-C3⁽ᴿᴬᵁ⁾
13 C3-P3⁽ᴿᴬᵁ⁾
14 P3-O1⁽ᴿᴬᵁ⁾

16 Fp2-F4⁽ᴿᴬᵁ⁾
17 F4-C4⁽ᴿᴬᵁ⁾
18 C4-P4⁽ᴿᴬᵁ⁾
19 P4-O2⁽ᴿᴬᵁ⁾

21 Fz-Cz⁽ᴿᴬᵁ⁾
22 Cz-Pz⁽ᴿᴬᵁ⁾
23 X1-X2⁽ᴿᴬᵁ⁾
61bpm

Figure 9.5(c) Emergence of epileptiform activity as anesthesia is tapered.

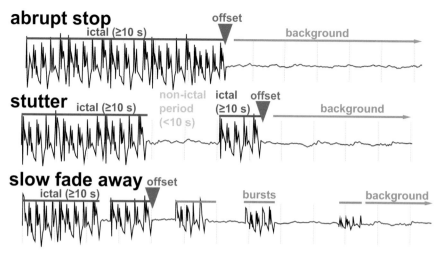

Figure 9.6 Patterns of SE cessation.

Absence SE

Case A 4-year-old girl presents with a few hours of inattention and "sluggishness" at school. Figure 9.7 shows a snapshot of her EEG.

How would you describe the EEG findings?
The EEG (Figure 9.7) shows continuous 3 Hz generalized spike-wave discharges.

What is your interpretation?
*These findings are consistent with **absence SE**.*

Absence SE consists of continuous (or repetitive) absence seizures for 30 minutes or longer. It manifests as impaired awareness with subtle motor automatisms that may last several hours or days. EEG shows continuous ~3 Hz generalized spike-wave discharges. Introduction or withdrawal of medications (especially benzodiazepines) and other toxic or metabolic disturbances are common triggers. A rapidly acting IV benzodiazepine (e.g., diazepam or lorazepam) is usually effective [11].

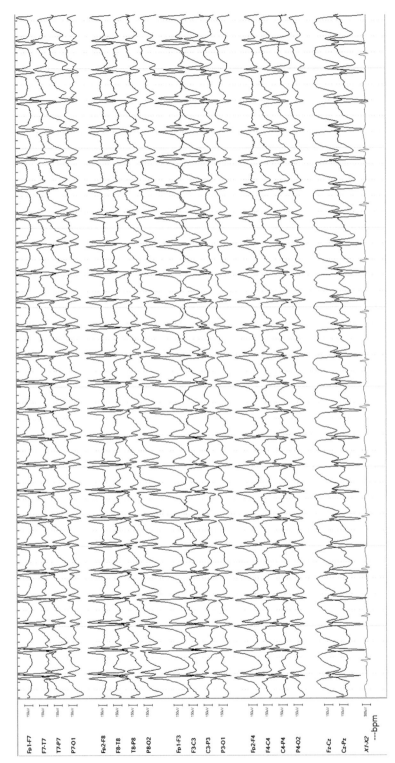

Figure 9.7 EEG of a patient presenting with inattention and "sluggishness" at school.

Case A 72-year-old woman presents with acute confusion and a history of chronic benzodiazepine use. Figure 9.8 shows a snapshot of her EEG.

How would you describe the EEG findings?
The EEG (Figure 9.8) shows continuous, fluctuating 3–4 Hz generalized spike-wave discharges consistent with NCSE.

What is your interpretation?
*In the present clinical context, these findings suggest **"de novo"** **absence SE**.*

De novo absence SE is a rare form of NCSE, often seen in older adults without a known diagnosis of epilepsy. It presents with acute onset of confusion, often in the setting of alcoholism and/or benzodiazepine use (or withdrawal). Continuous generalized spike-wave discharges are seen on EEG. Treatment with a broad-spectrum IV-ASM such as levetiracetam is often effective [12].

References

1. Leitinger M, Beniczky S, Rohracher A, et al. Salzburg consensus criteria for non-convulsive status epilepticus – Approach to clinical application. *Epilepsy & Behavior*. 2015 Aug 1;49:158–63.
2. Leitinger M, Trinka E, Zimmermann G, Beniczky S. Salzburg criteria for nonconvulsive status epilepticus: Details matter. *Epilepsia*. 2019 Nov;60(11):2334.
3. Krogstad MH, Høgenhaven H, Beier CP, Krøigård T. Nonconvulsive status epilepticus: Validating the Salzburg criteria against an expert EEG examiner. *Journal of Clinical Neurophysiology*. 2019 Mar 1;36(2):141–5.
4. Trinka E, Cock H, Hesdorffer D, et al. A definition and classification of status epilepticus: Report of the ILAE Task Force on Classification of Status Epilepticus. *Epilepsia*. 2015 Oct;56(10):1515–23.
5. Rossetti AO, Lowenstein DH. Management of refractory status epilepticus in adults: Still more questions than answers. *Lancet Neurology*. 2011 Oct 1;10 (10):922–30.
6. Hocker SE, Britton JW, Mandrekar JN, Wijdicks EF, Rabinstein AA. Predictors of outcome in refractory status epilepticus. *JAMA Neurology*. 2013 Jan 1;70(1):72–7.
7. Phabphal K, Chisurajinda S, Somboon T, Unwongse K, Geater A. Does burst suppression achieve seizure control in refractory status epilepticus? *BMC Neurology*. 2018 Dec;18(1):1–7.
8. Das AS, Lee JW, Izzy S, Vaitkevicius H. Ultra-short burst suppression as a "reset switch" for refractory status epilepticus. *Seizure: European Journal of Epilepsy*. 2019 Jan 1;64:41–4.
9. Johnson EL, Martinez NC, Ritzl EK. EEG characteristics of successful burst suppression for refractory status epilepticus. *Neurocritical Care*. 2016 Dec;25 (3):407–14.

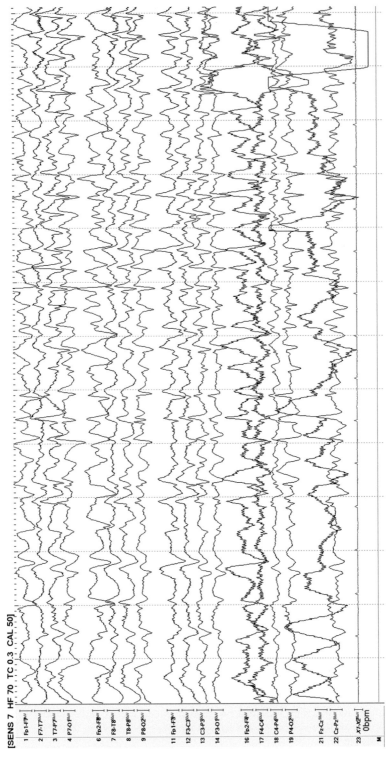

Figure 9.8 EEG of a patient presenting with acute confusion and a history of chronic benzodiazepine use.

10. Thompson SA, Hantus S. Highly epileptiform bursts are associated with seizure recurrence. *Journal of Clinical Neurophysiology.* 2016 Feb 1;33(1):66–71.

11. Panayiotopoulos CP. Typical absence seizures and their treatment. *Archives of Disease in Childhood.* 1999 Oct 1;81(4):351–5.

12. Datta P, Hope O, Kalamangalam GP. Teaching NeuroImages: De novo absence status epilepticus in an adult. *Neurology.* 2016 Apr 26;86(17):e186.

Learning Points
- Plus [+] terms
- Evolution
- Ictal-interictal continuum (IIC)

- Interictal (not ictal) patterns
- Stimulus induced (SI)
  patterns

Case A 52-year-old man with a history of alcoholism presents to the emergency room after multiple witnessed convulsions. Figure 10.1(a) shows a snapshot of his EEG.

How would you describe the EEG findings?
The EEG shows frequent right hemisphere LPDs. Additionally, fast activity is superimposed on each discharge.

What is your interpretation?
Superimposed fast activity is one type of plus [+] modifier that describes morphology. Hence, this pattern is called LPDs+F.

Another snapshot of the same patient's EEG shows the following pattern after treatment (Figure 10.1(b)).

How would you describe the EEG findings?
The EEG (Figure 10.1(b)) shows frequent right hemispheric LPDs with underlying rhythmic delta activity (RDA) associated with the discharges.

What is your interpretation?
Underlying RDA is another plus modifier. Hence, this pattern is called LPDs+R. Note that unlike lateralized spike and wave (LSW), here the spikes are not time-locked to the slow waves.

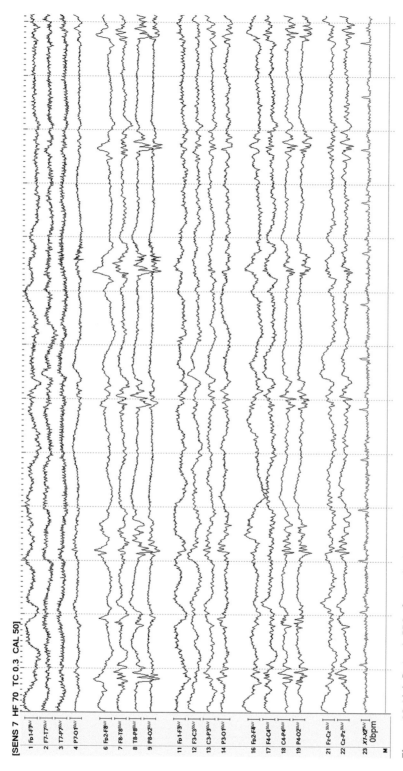

[SENS 7 HF 70 TC 0.3 CAL 50]

1 Fp1-F7
2 F7-T7
3 T7-P7
4 P7-O1

6 Fp2-F8
7 F8-T8
8 T8-P8
9 P8-O2

11 Fp1-F3
12 F3-C3
13 C3-P3
14 P3-O1

16 Fp2-F4
17 F4-C4
18 C4-P4
19 P4-O2

21 Fz-Cz
22 Cz-Pz
23 X1-X2
0bpm

Figure 10.1(a) Patient's EEG after multiple convulsive seizures.

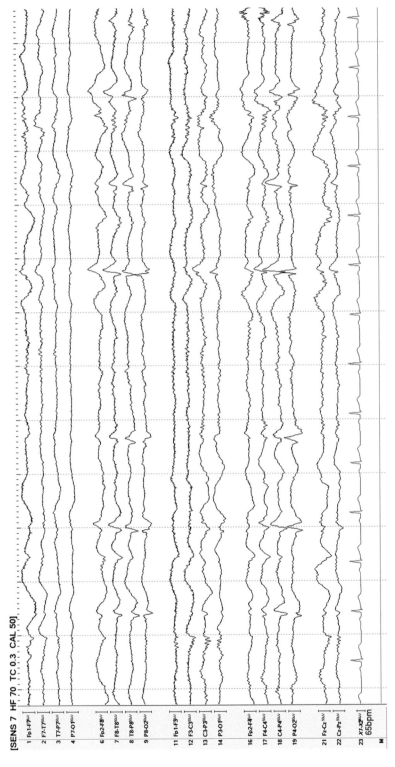

Figure 10.1(b) Patient's EEG after treatment.

Case A 28-year-old man with multiple sclerosis presents with generalized tonic clonic seizures. Figure 10.2 shows a snapshot of his EEG.

How would you describe the EEG findings?
The EEG shows left hemisphere LRDA. Additionally, there are sporadic embedded sharp waves, making this pattern LRDA+S.

What is your interpretation?
Superimposed sharply contoured activity including spikes or sharp waves is another plus modifier. This pattern is called LRDA+S. Again, the sharp or spike waves are not time-locked to the slow waves, differentiating this pattern from lateralized spike and wave (LSW).

Plus [+] Terms

As described previously, plus modifiers include superimposed fast activity (+F), spike/sharp waves (+S), or rhythmic delta activity (+R).

Though +F may be applied to both PDs and RDA, +R applies only to PDs, and +S only to RDA.

[+] modifiers may have the following electroclinical significance:

- A more epileptiform or ictal (seizure-like) appearance
- More likely to be associated with seizures
- More likely to show clinical and electrographic improvement if treated with IV-ASMs.

Hence [+] patterns are estimated to lie closer to the ictal end of the IIC.

Approach to management: If symptomatic (e.g., impaired awareness or focal neurological deficits), first try an IV benzodiazepine (e.g., lorazepam) or, alternatively, a loading dose of (non-benzodiazepine) IV-ASM. Observe for both clinical and EEG improvement.

Other individuals with [+] patterns are commonly treated with ASMs but the potential benefit of completely suppressing these patterns is unclear [1–3].

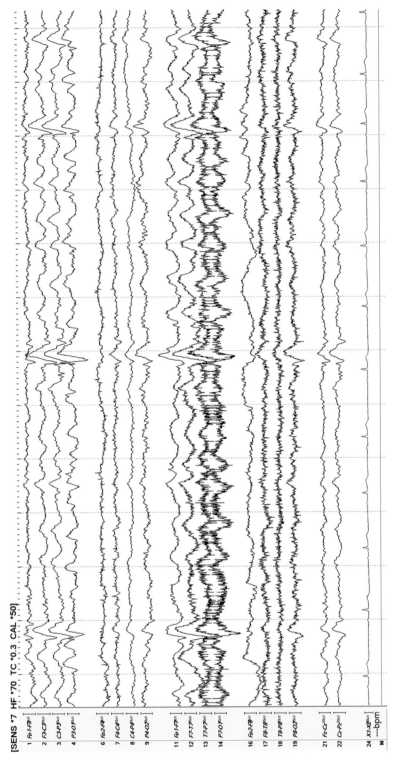

[SENS *7 HF *70 TC *0.3 CAL *50]

1 Fp1-F3⁵⁰ᵛ
2 F3-C3⁵⁰ᵛ
3 C3-P3⁵⁰ᵛ
4 P3-O1⁵⁰ᵛ

6 Fp2-F4⁵⁰ᵛ
7 F4-C4⁵⁰ᵛ
8 C4-P4⁵⁰ᵛ
9 P4-O2⁵⁰ᵛ

11 Fp1-F7⁵⁰ᵛ
12 F7-T7⁵⁰ᵛ
13 T7-P7⁵⁰ᵛ
14 P7-O1⁵⁰ᵛ

16 Fp2-F8⁵⁰ᵛ
17 F8-T8⁵⁰ᵛ
18 T8-P8⁵⁰ᵛ
19 P8-O2⁵⁰ᵛ

21 Fz-Cz⁵⁰ᵛ
22 Cz-Pz⁵⁰ᵛ

24 X1-X2⁵⁰ᵛ
M ---bpm

Figure 10.2 Patient's EEG after GTCs.

Case A 64-year-old man suddenly develops aphasia and confusion after a left craniotomy for subdural hematoma. Figures 10.3(a) and (b) show successive snapshots of his EEG.

How will you describe the EEG findings?

Figure 10.3(a) shows left hemispheric LPDs most prominent over the paracentral region. They are seen to increase from 1 to 2 Hz (change of frequency 1, i.e., 1 to 2 Hz). Next, in Figure 10.3(b), these LPDs have transformed to faster 3 Hz (change of frequency 2, i.e., 2 to 3 Hz). Each change is observed to persist for more than 3 cycles.

What is your interpretation?

These are evolving LPDs as they show two successive changes in frequency. Patterns may also show evolution in morphology and location as described in this section. Evolution is one of the electrographic hallmarks of ictal activity (seizures).

Evolving Patterns

Evolving patterns show *at least two* distinct changes in either frequency, morphology, or location with time.

- *Frequency*: The initial change in frequency should persist for at least 3 cycles followed by the second change of frequency which should again persist for at least another 3 cycles.
- *Morphology*: The initial change in morphology should persist for at least 3 cycles followed by the second change in morphology which should again persist for at least another 3 cycles.
- *Location*: The initial pattern must spread in or out in at least two electrodes with the involvement of each electrode location persisting for at least 3 cycles.

Though evolution requires at least two changes, each of which should persist for at least 3 cycles (occur three times continuously), however the changes should not be prolonged (less than 5 minutes).

Changes in voltage (amplitude) alone do not qualify as evolution. If an evolving pattern exceeds 4 Hz and lasts less than 10 seconds, it may qualify as a brief potentially ictal rhythmic discharge (BIRD); more on this later.

Fluctuating patterns are those which show at least three changes in frequency, morphology, or location that occur within 1 minute, but do not qualify as evolution. Most commonly, they include patterns with frequency fluctuations (same case, Figure 10.4), but they may also include patterns with alternating two morphologies or spreading in and out of a single additional electrode location.

Static patterns are those that do not evolve or fluctuate [1].

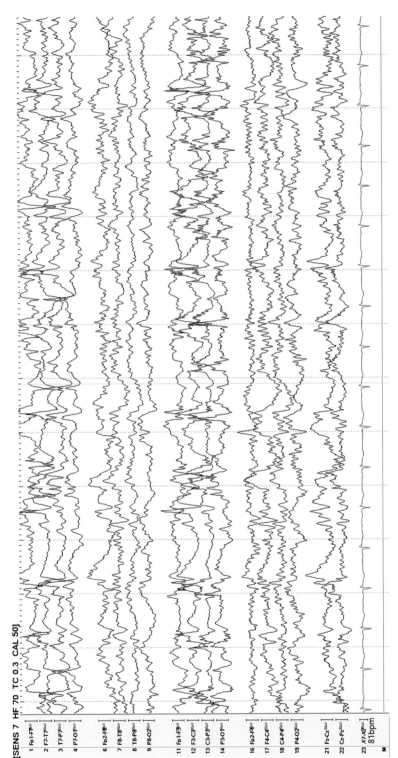

Figure 10.3(a) Patient's EEG with aphasia and confusion, page 1.

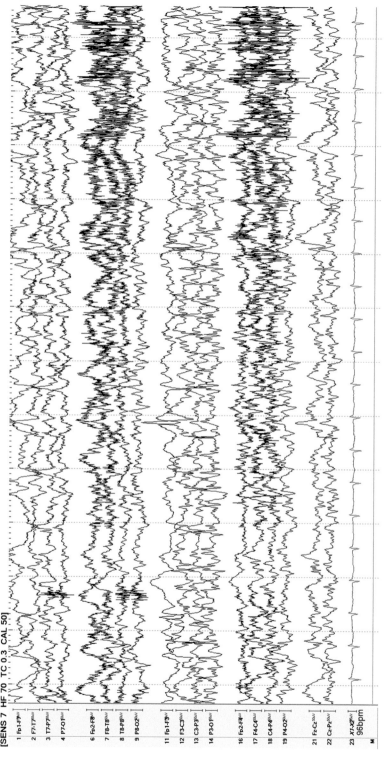

[SENS 7   HF 70   TC 0.3   CAL 50]

1 Fp1-F7⁵⁰ᵘⱽ
2 F7-T7⁵⁰ᵘⱽ
3 T7-P7⁵⁰ᵘⱽ
4 P7-O1⁵⁰ᵘⱽ
6 Fp2-F8⁵⁰ᵘⱽ
7 F8-T8⁵⁰ᵘⱽ
8 T8-P8⁵⁰ᵘⱽ
9 P8-O2⁵⁰ᵘⱽ
11 Fp1-F3⁵⁰ᵘⱽ
12 F3-C3⁵⁰ᵘⱽ
13 C3-P3⁵⁰ᵘⱽ
14 P3-O1⁵⁰ᵘⱽ
16 Fp2-F4⁵⁰ᵘⱽ
17 F4-C4⁵⁰ᵘⱽ
18 C4-P4⁵⁰ᵘⱽ
19 P4-O2⁵⁰ᵘⱽ
21 Fz-Cz⁵⁰ᵘⱽ
22 Cz-Pz⁵⁰ᵘⱽ
23 X1-X2⁵⁰ᵘⱽ
96bpm
M

Figure 10.3(b) Patient's EEG with aphasia and confusion, page 2.

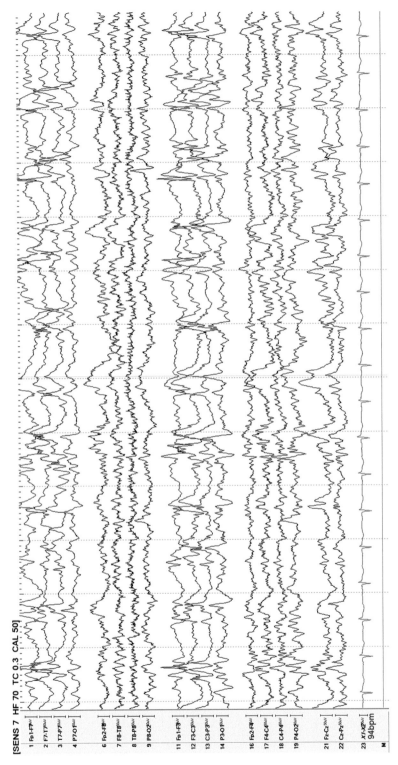

Figure 10.4 LPDs with frequency fluctuations.

Case, continued The 64-year-old patient described earlier is treated with IV lorazepam and loading doses of levetiracetam and valproate. He becomes sedated and further mental status assessment is challenging. Figure 10.5 shows a subsequent snapshot of his EEG.

How would you describe the EEG findings?
Figure 10.5 shows 0.5–1 Hz left hemispheric LPDs with fluctuation and superimposed fast activity (+F).

What is your interpretation?
This pattern lies on the ictal-interictal continuum (IIC). Even though it may not qualify as electrographic SE (<2.5 Hz, no evolution), it can potentially contribute to the patient's symptoms.

Ictal-Interictal Continuum (IIC)

Often, a pattern may not qualify as electrographic status epilepticus (ESE) or electrographic seizures (ESz) yet it contributes to neurological symptoms (e.g., impaired awareness). Such potentially ictal patterns lie on a continuum between definite NCSE and interictal (nonictal) patterns. Sometimes, they may be referred to as "possible" ESz/ESE.

Broadly, IIC patterns may include:

- Epileptic discharges (SW or PDs) between 2.5 and 1 Hz for over 10 seconds (i.e., 10–25 discharges in 10 seconds), or possibly even slower (1–0.5 Hz) but with plus modifiers or fluctuation; *or*
- Lateralized RDA (i.e., not GRDA) of $\geq$1 Hz for over 10 seconds (i.e., at least 10 slow waves in 10 seconds) with plus modifiers or fluctuation.

Importantly, the IIC is dynamic. Similar patterns may not only lie at opposite ends of the IIC in different patients, but they may also transition between the ictal-interictal extremes in the same patient or during the same recording.

Approach to management: A trial of treatment with an IV-ASM is often indicated given the ictal potential of IIC patterns. After treatment, a shift away from the ictal end of the continuum may be observed [1].

Interictal (Not Ictal) Patterns

Any PDs/lateralized RDA (i.e., not GRDA) of <2.5 Hz with relatively uniform morphology and no plus modifiers or fluctuations may be estimated to lie at the interictal end of the IIC.

Approach to management: These patterns may persist, depending on the underlying etiology. Antiseizure medication should be continued for seizure prevention, but the benefit of completely suppressing such patterns is unclear.

Figure 10.6 shows an example of persistent static LPDs in the 64-year-old patient after treatment.

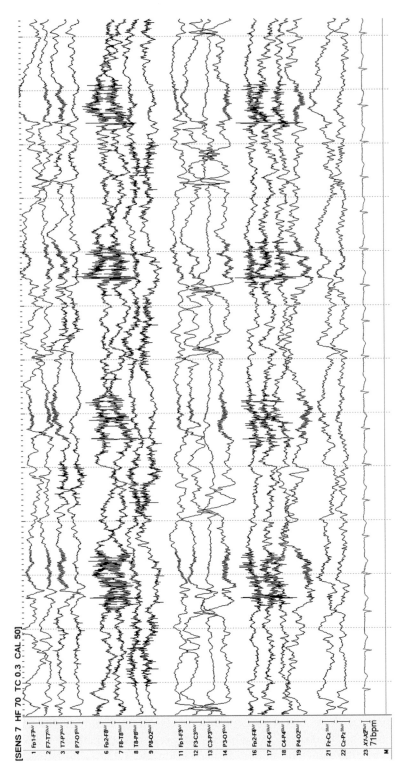

Figure 10.5 Patient's EEG after treatment.

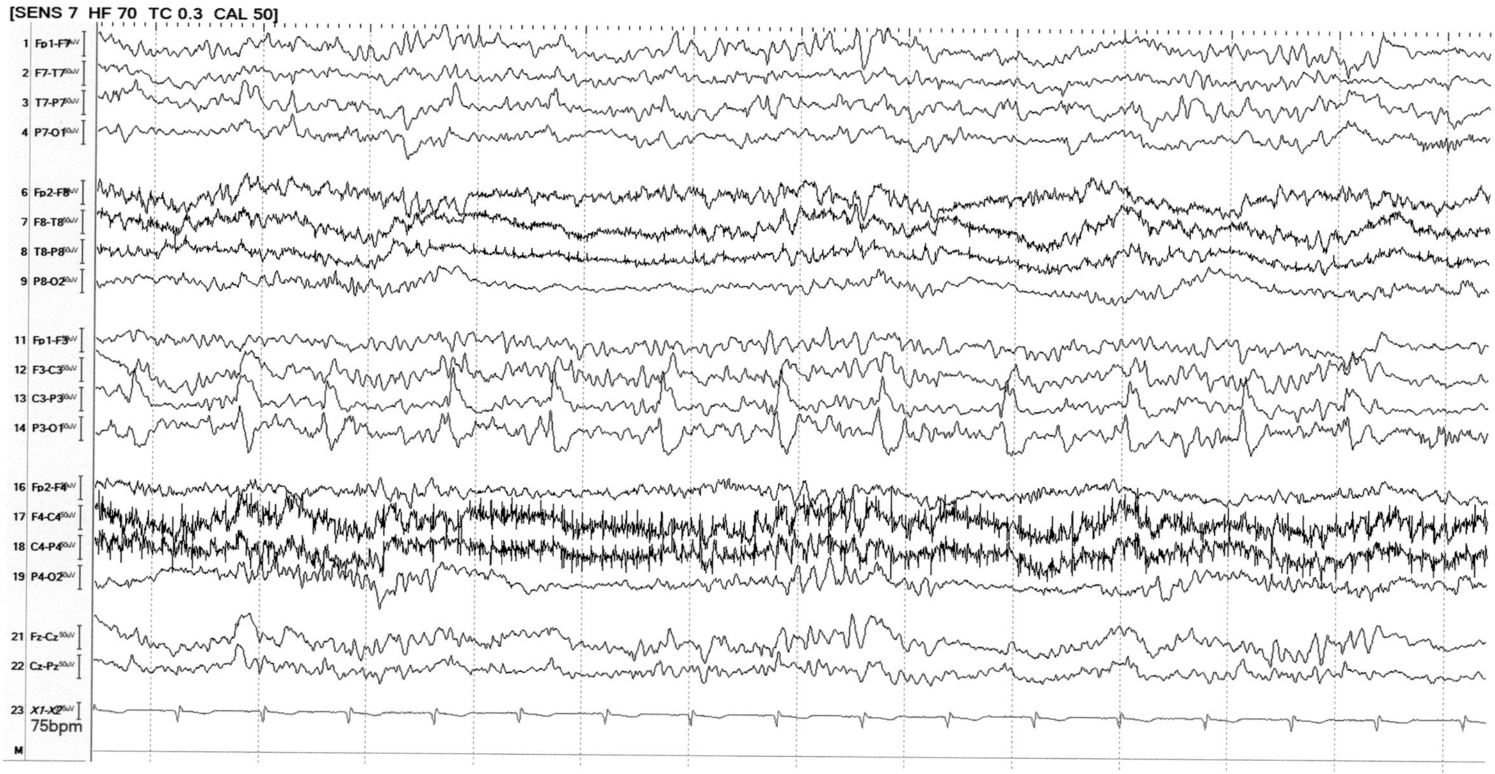
[SENS 7 HF 70 TC 0.3 CAL 50]
1 Fp1-F7
2 F7-T7
3 T7-P7
4 P7-O1
6 Fp2-F8
7 F8-T8
8 T8-P8
9 P8-O2
11 Fp1-F3
12 F3-C3
13 C3-P3
14 P3-O1
16 Fp2-F4
17 F4-C4
18 C4-P4
19 P4-O2
21 Fz-Cz
22 Cz-Pz
23 X1-X2
75bpm
M

Figure 10.6 Static LPDs.

Case An 83-year-old woman with Alzheimer dementia is being treated for a urinary tract infection. Figure 10.7(a) shows a snapshot of her baseline EEG, and Figure 10.7(b) shows a snapshot of her EEG during tactile stimulation.

How will you describe the EEG findings?
The baseline EEG (Figure 10.7(a)) shows a relatively organized but slow and low amplitude background with a few discharges with triphasic morphology. However, stimulation (Figure 10.7(b)) is associated with evolving GRDA+S.

What is your interpretation?
The above pattern is consistent with stimulus induced rhythmic, periodic, or ictal discharges (SIRPIDs).

Stimulus Induced Patterns

Stimulus induced (SI) patterns including rhythmic, periodic, or ictal discharges (SIRPIDs) occur in ~10% of critically ill patients. Stimulus induced seizures may also be observed. Sometimes, existing patterns may paradoxically terminate with stimulation (ST).

To qualify, a pattern should be reproduced or exacerbated by an alerting stimulus (even though the patient may not always clinically arouse).

The type of stimulus (e.g., auditory, light touch, regular clinical care, or other non-noxious or noxious stimuli) should be specified.

Approach to management: Stimulus induced patterns may be the result of abnormal (sometimes epileptogenic) arousals. Antiseizure medications may be used to treat epileptiform or ictal appearing patterns but the benefit of completely suppressing these waveforms is unclear [4,5].

References

1. Hirsch LJ, Fong MW, Leitinger M, et al. American Clinical Neurophysiology Society's Standardized Critical Care EEG Terminology: 2021 version. *Journal of Clinical Neurophysiology*. 2021 Jan 1;38(1):1.
2. Johnson EL, Kaplan PW. Population of the ictal-interictal injury zone: The significance of periodic and rhythmic activity. *Clinical Neurophysiology Practice*. 2017 Jan 1;2:107–18.
3. Gelisse P, Crespel A, Genton P, Jallon P, Kaplan PW. Lateralized periodic discharges: Which patterns are interictal injury, ictal, or peri-ictal? *Clinical Neurophysiology*. 2021 Jul 1;132(7):1593–603.

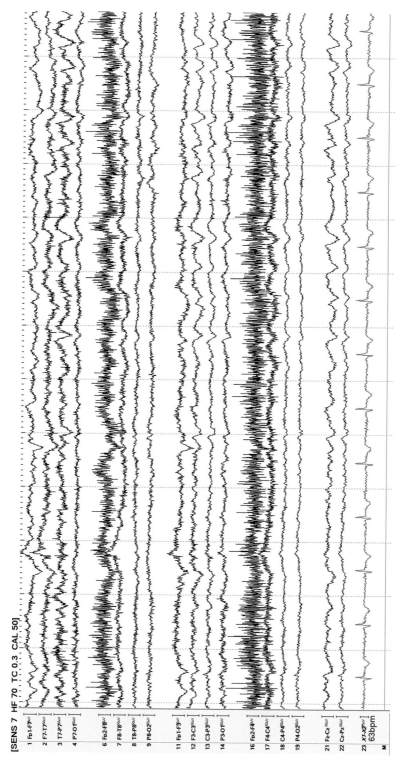

[SENS 7 HF 70 TC 0.3 CAL 50]

1 Fp1-F7^{50uV}
2 F7-T7^{50uV}
3 T7-P7^{50uV}
4 P7-O1^{50uV}
6 Fp2-F8^{50uV}
7 F8-T8^{50uV}
8 T8-P8^{50uV}
9 P8-O2^{50uV}
11 Fp1-F3^{50uV}
12 F3-C3^{50uV}
13 C3-P3^{50uV}
14 P3-O1^{50uV}
16 Fp2-F4^{50uV}
17 F4-C4^{50uV}
18 C4-P4^{50uV}
19 P4-O2^{50uV}
21 Fz-Cz^{50uV}
22 Cz-Pz^{50uV}
23 X1-X2^{50uV}
63bpm
M

Figure 10.7(a) Patient's EEG before stimulation.

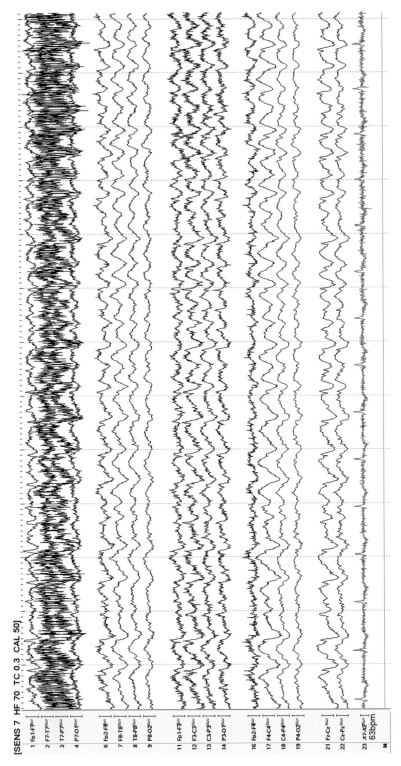

Figure 10.7(b) Patient's EEG after stimulation.

4. Hirsch LJ, Claassen J, Mayer SA, Emerson RG. Stimulus-induced rhythmic, periodic, or ictal discharges (SIRPIDs): A common EEG phenomenon in the critically ill. *Epilepsia.* 2004 Feb;45(2):109–23.

5. Braksick SA, Burkholder DB, Tsetsou S, et al. Associated factors and prognostic implications of stimulus-induced rhythmic, periodic, or ictal discharges. *JAMA Neurology.* 2016 May 1;73(5):585–90.

Chapter 11 — Seizures and Epileptiform Discharges

Learning Points
- Seizures
- Seizure burden

- Brief potentially ictal rhythmic discharges (BIRDs)
- Sporadic epileptiform discharges

Case A 68-year-old lady presents with altered mentation in the setting of pneumonia and sepsis. Figure 11.1 shows a snapshot of her EEG.

How would you describe the EEG findings?
The EEG (Figure 11.1) shows focal continuous ~4 Hz rhythmic sharp wave activity over the left hemisphere with a temporal predominance.

What is your interpretation?
This pattern of rhythmic sharp activity at a frequency of >2.5 Hz for a duration of 10 seconds is consistent with electrographic seizure.

Seizures

Electrographic seizures (ESz) are patterns of 10 seconds or longer and characterized by either:

- Epileptic discharges (spikes, sharps, or sharply contoured activity) of >2.5 Hz, *or*
- Other patterns with definite evolution.

Here, the "10 second" limit is purely by convention.

If these patterns are associated with a clinical correlate (e.g., gaze deviation, eye movements, facial or limb twitching), they are instead called **electroclinical seizures (ECSz)**, even if <10 seconds in duration.

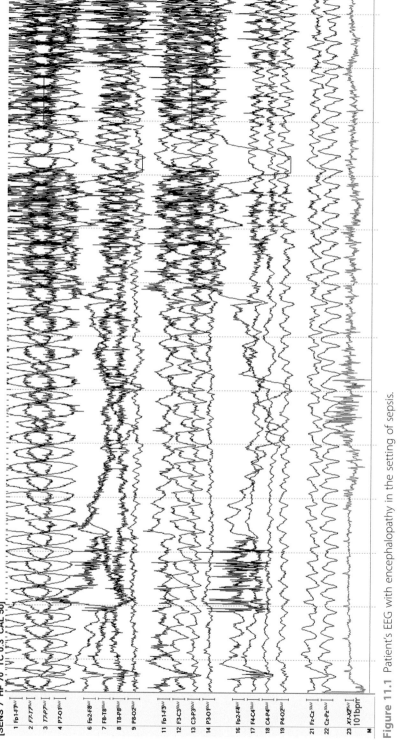

Figure 11.1 Patient's EEG with encephalopathy in the setting of sepsis.

Additionally, many seizures may classify as both electrographic and electroclinical; also both types may occur in the same patient or during the same EEG recording [1,2].

Seizure Burden

An hourly (or daily) seizure burden should be estimated with CEEG monitoring.

- This may be calculated as the total duration of seizure activity (or other ictal patterns) per hour. For example, 10 60-second-long seizures in one hour would mean a seizure burden of 10 minutes.

Approach to management: Seizure burden of >12 minutes per hour (i.e., >20%) may be associated with neurological decline. In these patients, early escalation of antiseizure treatments may be useful [2,3].

Case A 73-year-old man with traumatic brain injury, spastic quadriplegia, and chronic drug resistant epilepsy who presented with breakthrough seizures after a urinary tract infection. Figure 11.2 shows a snapshot of his EEG.

How would you describe the EEG findings?
The EEG (Figure 11.2) shows approximately 7-second-long runs of focal evolving rhythmic discharges of >4 Hz over the right temporal region. There is no associated clinical correlate that can be identified at the bedside.

What is your interpretation?
This pattern of evolving rhythmic sharp activity at a frequency of >2.5 Hz does not qualify as an electrographic seizure because of the absence of an apparent clinical correlate and a duration of less than 10 seconds.

Instead, the appropriate description should be a focal brief potentially ictal rhythmic discharge (BIRD).

Brief Potentially Ictal Rhythmic Discharges (BIRDs)

These are brief runs of focal, lateralized, or generalized rhythmic activity (or paroxysmal fast activity) that are too short to qualify as electrographic seizures despite their ictal appearance. They are not associated with obvious clinical symptoms.

They have the following electrographic characteristics:

- Frequency of >4 Hz
- Duration between 0.5 and 10 seconds

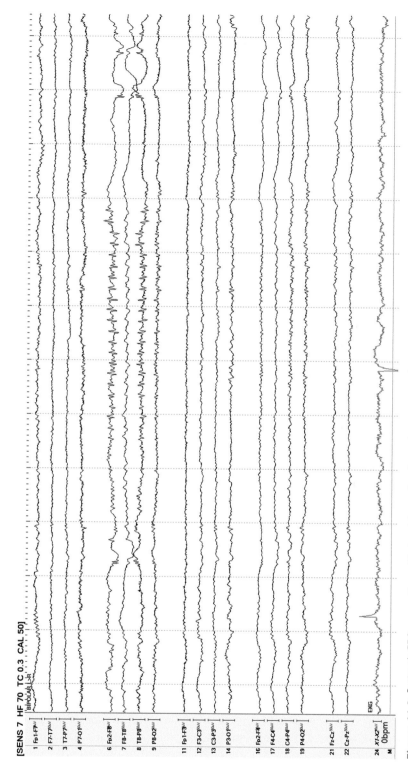

Figure 11.2 Patient's EEG, presenting with breakthrough seizures in a setting of traumatic brain injury and UTI.

- Definite BIRDs: Similar location and morphology to previously known epileptiform discharges or seizures, or clear evolution.

Significance: These occur in both critically ill and non-critically ill patients.

- Acute brain injuries: BIRDs commonly occur along with other ictal and interictal patterns (e.g., LPDs and/or seizures).
- Epilepsy: In those not critically ill, they are associated with refractory epilepsy.

Of note, normal patterns (e.g., arousals), benign variants, or bursts (as in burst-suppression or burst-attenuation) may be misidentified as BIRDs.

Approach to management: By definition, BIRDs are asymptomatic (if symptomatic, they qualify as seizures). However, given their ictal potential and association with seizure risk, they should be treated with ASMs for further seizure prevention [2,4,5]. In fact, BIRDs may be a scalp EEG biomarker of ictal activity that is only detectable with intracranial recording [5].

Case A 25-year-old lady with a left temporal mass status post resection and subsequent drug resistant epilepsy. Figure 11.3 shows a snapshot of her EEG.

How would you describe the EEG findings?
The EEG (Figure 11.3) shows multiple focal sharp waves predominantly over the left temporal region (F7/T7 electrodes) during sleep.

What is your interpretation?
The finding of sleep accentuated right temporal sharp waves (epileptiform discharges) is consistent with the interictal manifestations of a focal epilepsy disorder in the above clinical context.

Sporadic Epileptiform Discharges

Sporadic epileptiform discharges are abnormal transient waves with pointed morphologies that distinctly stand out from the baseline electrographic activity and are associated with risk for epileptic seizures.

They occur sporadically, either as isolated discharges or brief trains, but do not occur with a consistent frequency, i.e., they are not rhythmic or periodic.

Depending on their duration (base), they are called **spikes** (20–70 milliseconds) or **sharps** (70–200 milliseconds). Often, there is also an aftercoming slow wave (spike and wave, or spike-wave). If multiple spikes occur together, they are called polyspikes.

Despite sharps and spikes having slightly different morphologies, both these patterns have the same clinical significance – they are associated with epileptic seizure risk, hence they are called "epileptiform discharges."

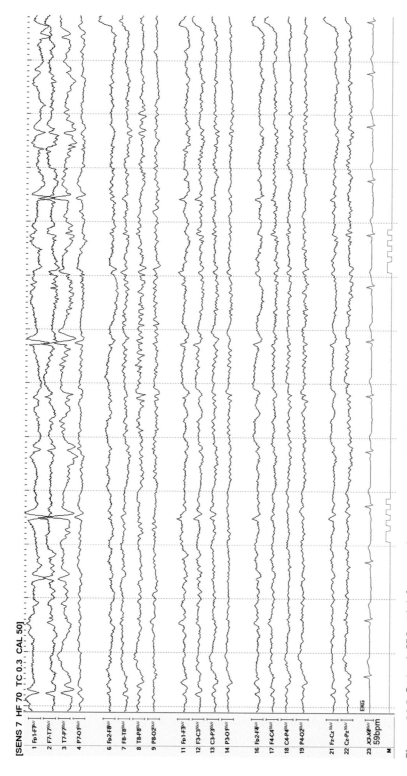

Figure 11.3 Patient's EEG with left temporal mass complicated by focal epilepsy.

Types

- Focal: spike or sharp waves that predominate over a single hemisphere. They can be seen with focal epilepsy.
- Generalized: spike or sharp waves that occur symmetrically over both hemispheres. They can be seen with generalized epilepsy (Figure 11.4).

Case A 14-year-old boy with frequent myoclonic jerking presents to the emergency room after a first-time generalized tonic clonic seizure. Figure 11.4 shows a snapshot of his EEG.

How would you describe the EEG findings?
The EEG (Figure 11.4) shows brief bursts of frontally predominant ~ 3–4 Hz generalized spike and wave (GSW) discharges.

What is your interpretation?
Findings of generalized spike-wave discharges are consistent with the interictal manifestations of a generalized epilepsy disorder in the given clinical context.

Clinical Significance

Epilepsy is a clinical diagnosis; it refers to a condition of recurrent and unprovoked seizures. A single routine EEG has a relatively low sensitivity to detect epileptiform discharges in epilepsy (~30%). If epileptiform discharges are seen, then the EEG is more specific (78–98%) for the diagnosis of epilepsy. Though the finding of epileptiform discharges after an apparent first-time seizure may support the diagnosis of epilepsy, it is not necessarily confirmatory.

Rarely, epileptic discharges may occur without epilepsy:

- Approximately 1–5% of otherwise healthy individuals may have epileptic discharges on EEG.
- They may occur after acute or progressive cerebral disease or injury (e.g., bleeds, strokes, trauma, or tumors). Here, they can be associated with acute or symptomatic seizures.
- They may also occur in those with chronic cerebral disorders such as autism spectrum disorder (ASD), intellectual disability (ID), and Alzheimer disease (AD).

Approach to management: Most patients with epileptic discharges require antiseizure medications for seizure prevention. However, the benefit of treating asymptomatic epileptic discharges is unclear [6–8].

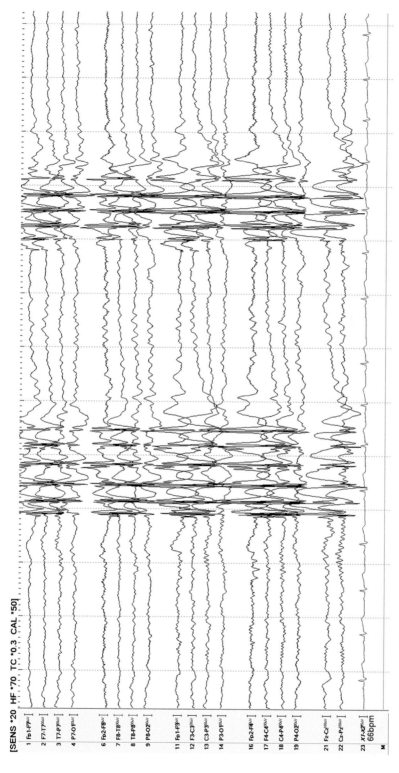

Figure 11.4 Patient's EEG, presenting with frequent body jerks.

References

1. Laccheo I, Sonmezturk H, Bhatt AB, et al. Non-convulsive status epilepticus and non-convulsive seizures in neurological ICU patients. *Neurocritical Care.* 2015 Apr;22(2):202–11.
2. Hirsch LJ, Fong MW, Leitinger M, et al. American Clinical Neurophysiology Society's Standardized Critical Care EEG Terminology: 2021 version. *Journal of Clinical Neurophysiology.* 2021 Jan 1;38(1):1.
3. Payne ET, Zhao XY, Frndova H, et al. Seizure burden is independently associated with short term outcome in critically ill children. *Brain.* 2014 May 1;137(5):1429–38.
4. Yoo JY, Rampal N, Petroff OA, Hirsch LJ, Gaspard N. Brief potentially ictal rhythmic discharges in critically ill adults. *JAMA Neurology.* 2014 Apr 1;71 (4):454–62.
5. Yoo JY, Jetté N, Kwon CS, et al. Brief potentially ictal rhythmic discharges and paroxysmal fast activity as scalp electroencephalographic biomarkers of seizure activity and seizure onset zone. *Epilepsia.* 2021 Mar;62(3):742–51.
6. Smith SJ. EEG in the diagnosis, classification, and management of patients with epilepsy. *Journal of Neurology, Neurosurgery & Psychiatry.* 2005 Jun 1;76(suppl 2): ii2–7.
7. Sam MC, So EL. Significance of epileptiform discharges in patients without epilepsy in the community. *Epilepsia.* 2001 Oct 29;42(10):1273–8.
8. Sanchez Fernandez I, Loddenkemper T, Galanopoulou AS, Moshé SL. Should epileptiform discharges be treated? *Epilepsia.* 2015 Oct;56(10):1492–504.

Chapter

12

Seizure Mimics

Learning Points
- Tremors
- Myoclonus

- Syncope
- Functional seizures/psychogenic non-epileptic seizures (PNES)

Case A 56-year-old man with a history of schizophrenia and long-standing neuroleptic use is admitted to the intensive care unit for management of heart failure. On examination, he is confused and has continuous right arm shaking. Figure 12.1 shows a snapshot of his EEG.

How would you describe the EEG findings?
> The EEG (Figure 12.1) shows a prominent continuous spiky ~5 Hz periodic pattern over the posterior head region.

What is your interpretation?
> Despite its sharp or spiky appearance, this rhythmic/periodic appearing myogenic artifact can be distinguished from true cerebral activity such as epileptiform discharges by the lack of a definite "field" and stereotyped appearance without evolution or fluctuation.
>
> Further, a correlation with ipsilateral arm shaking identifies this activity as tremor artifact.

Tremors

Tremors are involuntary rhythmic or oscillatory movements that commonly involve the head or extremities. Tremors of Parkinson disease or drug-induced parkinsonism (neuroleptics, metoclopramide, and phenothiazines) predominate at rest. However, those of alcohol withdrawal, neuropathy, or essential tremor (ET) are induced by postures or action. Tremors may mimic epileptic seizures in critically ill individuals.

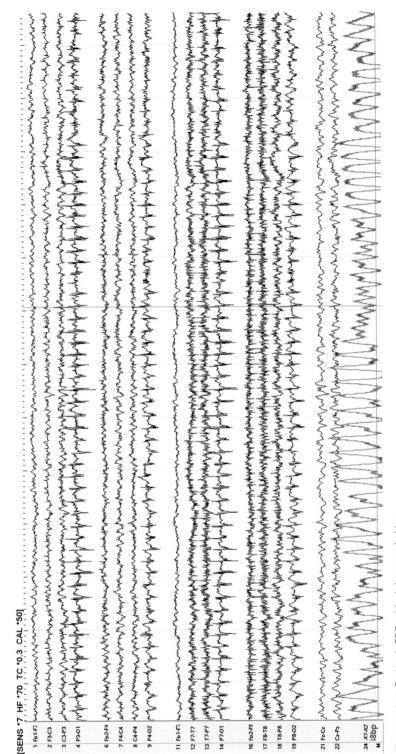

[SENS *7 HF *70 TC *0.3 CAL *50]

1 Fp1-F3
2 F3-C3
3 C3-P3
4 P3-O1

6 Fp2-F4
7 F4-C4
8 C4-P4
9 P4-O2

11 Fp1-F7
12 F7-T7
13 T7-P7
14 P7-O1

16 Fp2-F8
17 F8-T8
18 T8-P8
19 P8-O2

21 Fz-Cz
22 Cz-Pz

24 X1-X2
M |8bp

Figure 12.1 Patient's EEG with right arm shaking.

Similarly, a variety of other abnormal or involuntary movements such as posturing, rigors, shivering, or twitching are also common in critically ill patients. These abnormal or involuntary movements may also be distinguished from epileptic seizures by their characteristic pattern of myogenic artifact that clinically correlates with the motor activity at the bedside in the absence of epileptic activity on CEEG [1].

Case A 75-year-old woman with a history of COPD, atrial fibrillation, dementia, hypertension, hyperlipidemia, and depression presents to the emergency room after a witnessed cardiac arrest with return of spontaneous circulation following a single round of CPR. She is intubated and sedated on arrival. At the bedside, she is noted to have repetitive whole-body jerking movements. Figure 12.2 shows a snapshot of her EEG.

How would you describe the EEG findings?
The EEG (Figure 12.2) shows generalized delta and theta slowing without definite epileptiform discharges. Further, there are overlying bursts of low voltage EMG artifact corresponding to the jerking movements.

What is your interpretation?
The above electroclinical pattern is consistent with subcortical myoclonus. Myoclonic jerking and corresponding myogenic artifact are not associated with epileptiform discharges on EEG.

Case An 18-year-old man with a history of depression presents to the emergency room after a witnessed cardiac arrest secondary to a drug overdose with return of spontaneous circulation following multiple rounds of CPR. He is intubated in the field. At the bedside, he is comatose and has repetitive whole-body jerking movements. Figure 12.3 shows a snapshot of his EEG.

How would you describe the EEG findings?
The EEG (Figure 12.3) shows 1 Hz generalized periodic discharges (GPDs) associated with a brief high amplitude myogenic artifact. The discharges are best appreciated in the central channels (Fz-Cz, Cz-Pz) where scalp musculature is absent.

What is your interpretation?
The above electroclinical pattern is consistent with cortical myoclonus. Here, myoclonic jerking and corresponding myogenic artifact are associated with epileptiform discharges (jerks are time-locked to the discharges).

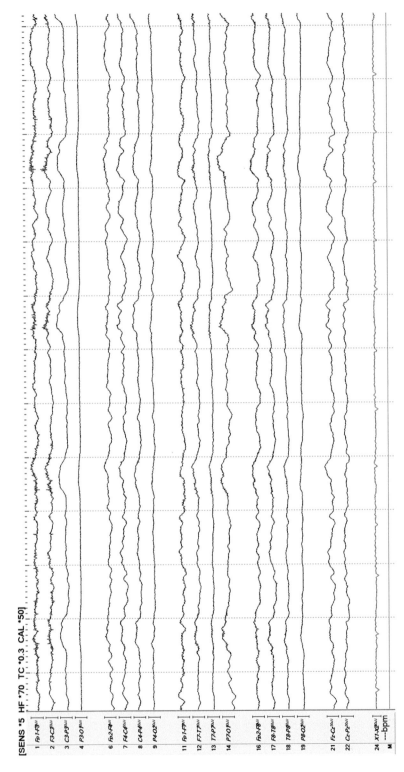

Figure 12.2 Patient's EEG after cardiac arrest.

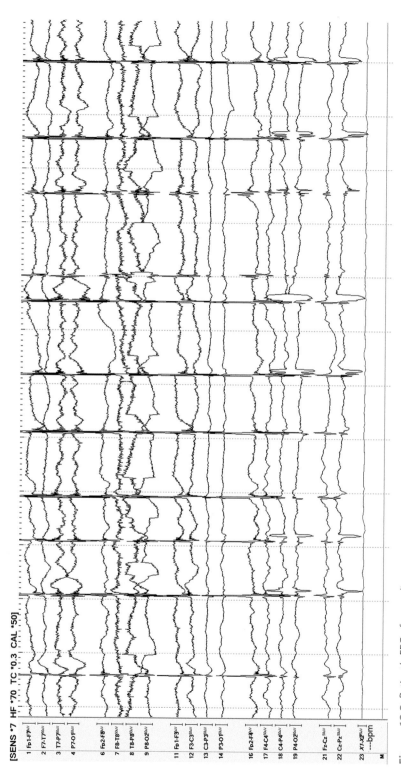

Figure 12.3 Patient's EEG after cardiac arrest.

Myoclonus

Myoclonus is another type of involuntary movement commonly encountered in critical illness. It manifests as a sudden brief increase (positive) or paradoxical loss (negative) of muscle tone resulting in focal or generalized, often repetitive, twitches or jerks.

There may be several potential etiologies of myoclonus in critically ill patients, such as drugs, infections, metabolic abnormalities, and/or cerebral hypoxia following cardiac arrest, affecting both the cortical or subcortical (including spinal and peripheral) neuroanatomical levels. However, cortical myoclonus may progress to frank epileptic seizures or status epilepticus and therefore should be recognized and treated with antiseizure medications such as levetiracetam, valproate, or clonazepam.

Cortical myoclonus is identified by the presence of generalized epileptiform discharges associated with the myoclonic jerk artifact (jerk-linked discharges). These are absent in myoclonus that is generated subcortically.

Rarely, EEG-EMG polygraphy may be used to confirm jerk-linked discharges [2].

Case A 53-year-old woman with ischemic heart disease is admitted for a bout of colitis. She is monitored on CEEG for "convulsions" further described as transient loss of consciousness and whole-body jerking. She experiences one such event while straining for a stool sample. Figures 12.4 (a–d) show successive snapshots of her EEG during this event.

How would you describe the EEG findings?
The EEGs above show the following electroclinical sequence of events during this patient's episode of transient loss of consciousness:

- *Figure 12.4(a) Normal waking background; however, acute onset of bradycardia noted on single ECG channel.*
- *Figure 12.4(b) Severe bradycardia on ECG is followed by diffuse slowing and attenuation of the electrographic background. She reports feeling lightheaded.*
- *Figure 12.4(c) Cardiac asystole on ECG and generalized suppression of the electrographic background. She experiences a transient loss of consciousness. A few jerking movements of her extremities are observed.*
- *Figure 12.4(d) Heart rate recovers, there is emergence of diffuse slowing followed by rapid restoration of electrographic background. She promptly recovers consciousness.*

What is your interpretation?
The above electroclinical sequence of ECG followed by EEG changes and corresponding transient loss of consciousness observed at the bedside is consistent with vasovagal syncope. Myoclonic jerks are common during syncope (convulsive syncope), often mimicking generalized tonic clonic seizures.

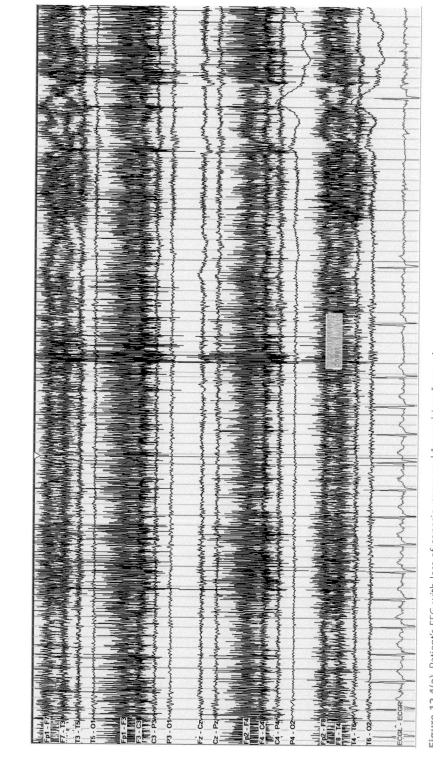

Figure 12.4(a) Patient's EEG with loss of consciousness and "convulsions," page 1.

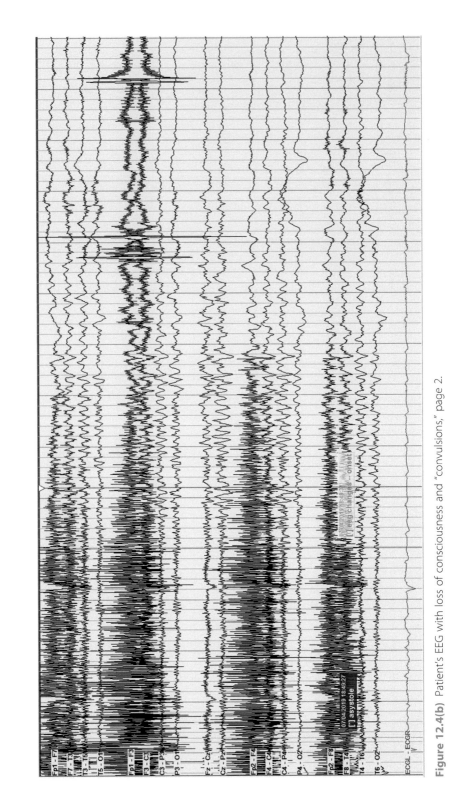

Figure 12.4(b) Patient's EEG with loss of consciousness and "convulsions," page 2.

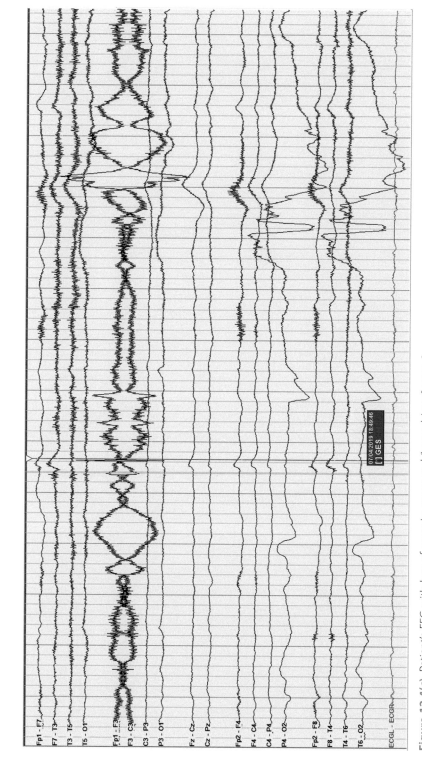

Figure 12.4(c) Patient's EEG with loss of consciousness and "convulsions," page 3.

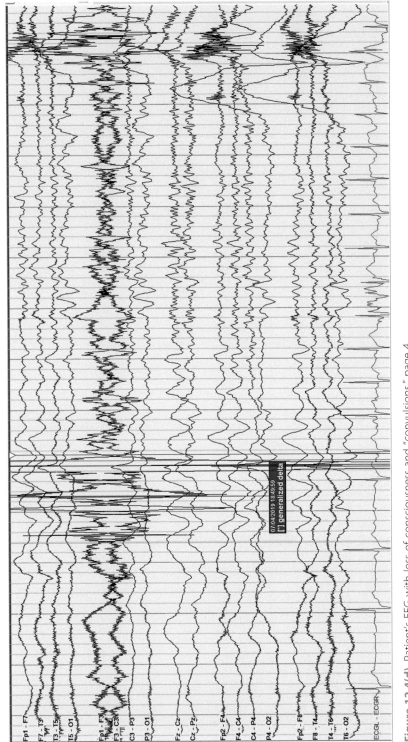

Figure 12.4(d) Patient's EEG with loss of consciousness and "convulsions," page 4.

Syncope

Syncope is defined as the transient loss of consciousness and postural tone due to a sudden impairment of cerebral blood flow to the brain. If it occurs due to increased vagal tone (bradycardia and hypotension), it is called vasovagal (neurocardiogenic) syncope. Investigation with tilt table testing may be useful. Less commonly, the etiology may be purely cardiac or neurogenic [3].

Case An 18-year-old woman with anxiety and bipolar disorder presents to the emergency room with multiple generalized convulsions. She is treated with intravenous lorazepam and loaded with antiseizure medication. Figure 12.5 shows a snapshot of her EEG during one such convulsive event.

How would you describe the EEG findings?

The EEG (Figure 12.5) shows excessive movement and myogenic artifact that may have a rhythmic appearance which obscures most of the recording. However, features of a normal waking background such as a posterior dominant rhythm are appreciated intermittently during the event.

What is your interpretation?

The presence of a normal waking background (including posterior dominant rhythm) in the setting of clinically apparent unresponsiveness is consistent with a diagnosis of functional/psychogenic non-epileptic seizure-like activity.

Functional Seizures/Psychogenic Non-Epileptic Seizures (PNES)

Known widely as psychogenic non-epileptic seizures (previously, "pseudo seizures"), **functional seizures** are a common mimic of true epileptic seizures, and prolonged episodes ("psychogenic status epilepticus") may result in unnecessary and potentially harmful interventions such as intubation, sedation, and antiseizure medication therapies. Functional seizures are commonly of longer duration (>3 minutes) and show fluctuating evolution compared to epileptic seizures. Other commonly reported ictal features that suggest a potentially functional/psychogenic (vs. epileptic) etiology include eye closure, side-to-side head movements, out of phase (asynchronous or opposite directions) limb movements, opisthotonos and/or intense rotational body movements, pelvic thrusting, and directed rage (kicking, punching, or thrashing). Vocalizations may include comprehensible words and memory recollections. During the postictal phase, most patients retain the ability to protect themselves from injury, such as avoidance of a falling arm. Tongue bite, urinary and/or fecal incontinence, and fall-related injuries are usually absent. Less commonly, both epileptic and functional seizures may coexist in the same patient.

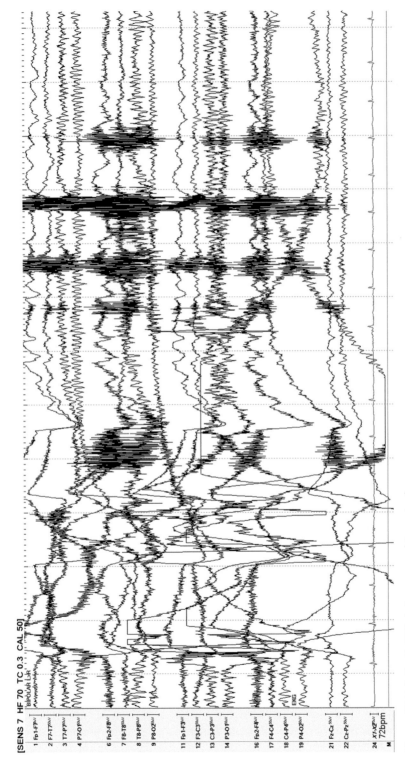

Figure 12.5 Patient's EEG during a convulsive episode.

Rarely, frontal lobe epileptic seizures may mimic functional seizures. Video-EEG monitoring with capture and characterization of the event in question may clarify the diagnosis [4].

References

1. Herman ST, Abend NS, Bleck TP, et al. Consensus statement on continuous EEG in critically ill adults and children, Part I: Indications. *Journal of Clinical Neurophysiology.* 2015 Apr;32(2):87.
2. Sutter R, Ristic A, Rüegg S, Fuhr P. Myoclonus in the critically ill: Diagnosis, management, and clinical impact. *Clinical Neurophysiology.* 2016 Jan 1;127(1): 67–80.
3. Brenner RP. Electroencephalography in syncope. *Journal of Clinical Neurophysiology.* 1997 May 1;14(3):197–209.
4. Oto M, Reuber M. Psychogenic non-epileptic seizures: Aetiology, diagnosis, and management. *Advances in Psychiatric Treatment.* 2014 Jan;20(1):13–22.

13

Learning Points
- Focal cerebral dysfunction
- Breach effect

- Lateralized rhythmic delta activity (LRDA)
- Epilepsia partialis continua (EPC)

Case A 70-year-old woman with valvular heart disease on warfarin presents with a left subdural hemorrhage after a fall. She is monitored on CEEG for episodes of confusion. Figure 13.1 shows a snapshot of her EEG.

How would you describe the EEG findings?

The EEG (Figure 13.1) shows focal voltage attenuation (reduced amplitude) of electrographic activity over the left hemisphere channels.

What is your interpretation?

Focal attenuation may be regional (e.g., frontal, temporal, or posterior) or hemispheric (e.g., right, left, or both hemispheres). It suggests underlying cortical neuronal dysfunction and/or increased impedance between the recording electrode and cortical surface, which may occur from a subcutaneous or subdural collection of blood, fluid, or pus, among other causes.

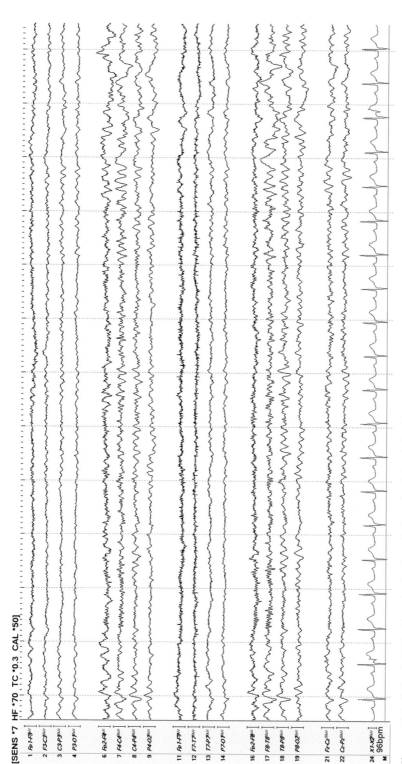

Figure 13.1 Patient's EEG with episode of confusion after left subdural hematoma.

Case: A 48-year-old man with chronic alcoholism presented with acute onset headache, aphasia, and dense hemiparesis. Head CT revealed a large left putaminal hemorrhage. He was monitored on CEEG for suspected seizures. Figure 13.2 shows a snapshot of his EEG.

How would you describe the EEG findings?
The EEG (Figure 13.2) shows focal polymorphic delta and theta activity (slow waves) over the left hemisphere channels.

What is your interpretation?
Focal slowing (regional or hemispheric) is also suggestive of underlying cortical neuronal dysfunction. This finding is not specific to an etiology but, rather, it estimates the location of the underlying cortical dysfunction.

Focal Cerebral Dysfunction

Focal attenuation and/or slowing suggests focal cortical neuronal dysfunction. This may occur due to the following causes:

- Structural problem – e.g., stroke, bleed, tumor, or abscess
- Physiological problem – e.g., postictal, ischemia, or migraine.

Structural lesions may be evident on neuroimaging (Head CT or Brain MRI); however, if these are absent, purely physiological etiologies may be considered as the cause of focal dysfunction. These sometimes require additional dedicated techniques to elucidate including metabolic, nuclear, or vascular studies. Frequently, both structural and physiological mechanisms may occur simultaneously in the same region.

Additionally, the reader should look carefully for focal epileptiform abnormalities such as epileptiform discharges, LPDs, or LRDA that indicate coexisting focal cortical irritability (increased seizure risk) [1].

Case A 49-year-old woman with a history of a right middle cerebral artery aneurysm status post craniotomy is admitted for multiple convulsive events. Figure 13.3 shows a snapshot of her EEG.

How would you describe the EEG findings?
The EEG (Figure 13.3) shows higher amplitudes, faster frequencies, and sharper morphologies of the background electrographic activity over the right hemisphere (especially the parasagittal electrodes Fp2, F4, C4, P4, and O2).

What is your interpretation?
This is consistent with breach effect in the setting of known right sided craniotomy.

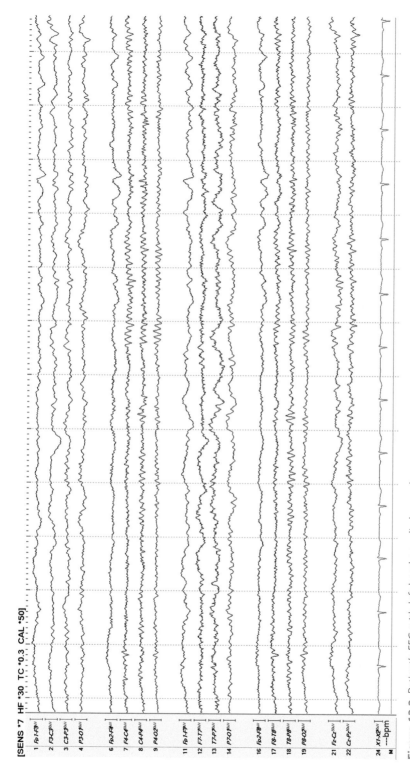

[SENS *7   HF *30   TC *0.3   CAL *50]

1 Fp1-F3⁵⁰ᵘᵛ
2 F3-C3⁵⁰ᵘᵛ
3 C3-P3⁵⁰ᵘᵛ
4 P3-O1⁵⁰ᵘᵛ

6 Fp2-F4⁵⁰ᵘᵛ
7 F4-C4⁵⁰ᵘᵛ
8 C4-P4⁵⁰ᵘᵛ
9 P4-O2⁵⁰ᵘᵛ

11 Fp1-F7⁵⁰ᵘᵛ
12 F7-T7⁵⁰ᵘᵛ
13 T7-P7⁵⁰ᵘᵛ
14 P7-O1⁵⁰ᵘᵛ

16 Fp2-F8⁵⁰ᵘᵛ
17 F8-T8⁵⁰ᵘᵛ
18 T8-P8⁵⁰ᵘᵛ
19 P8-O2⁵⁰ᵘᵛ

21 Fz-Cz⁵⁰ᵘᵛ
22 Cz-Pz⁵⁰ᵘᵛ

24 X1-X2⁵⁰ᵘᵛ
M ---bpm

Figure 13.2 Patient's EEG with left basal ganglia hemorrhage.

[SENS 7 HF 70 TC 0.3 CAL 50]

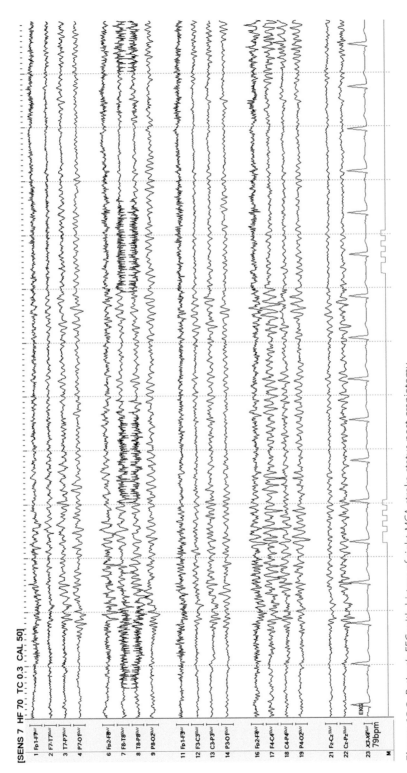

Figure 13.3 Patient's EEG with history of right MCA stroke status post craniotomy.

Breach Effect

This results from the loss of the normal dampening effect of skull bones on electrographic activity generated by cortical neurons and recorded by scalp electrodes. As a result, the background electrographic activity may show higher amplitudes, sharper morphologies, and/or excess faster frequencies over the focal region of missing bone. Breach effect may occur after craniotomy, skull fracture, or bone metastasis [2].

Case A 68-year-old woman with vascular risk factors is admitted for an episode of transient altered mentation and right sided weakness. Emergent CT head is normal. Figure 13.4 shows a snapshot of her EEG.

How would you describe the EEG findings?
The EEG (Figure 13.4) shows focal left temporal ~1 Hz monomorphic delta activity.

What is your interpretation?
Lateralized rhythmic delta activity.

Lateralized Rhythmic Delta Activity (LRDA)

This pattern of focal rhythmic delta slowing (even in the absence of [+] features) is common in critically ill patients and is associated with increased seizure risk (like LPDs). Seizures may be purely electrographic. Associated cortical or juxtacortical structural lesions may be detected on neuroimaging. As LRDA indicates focal cortical irritability (seizure risk), treatment with antiseizure medications is indicated for seizure prevention [3].

Case A 59-year-old woman with a right frontal meningioma presents with constant repetitive left arm jerking. A Head CT performed in the emergency room shows significant perilesional edema. Figure 13.5 shows a snapshot of her EEG.

How would you describe the EEG findings?
The EEG (Figure 13.5) shows blunted LPDs occurring at about 1 Hz over the right parasagittal region (maximal at C4). These waveforms clinically correlate with left arm jerking noted at the bedside.

What is your interpretation?
This electroclinical pattern of repetitive discharges time-locked to constant jerking movements noted at the bedside is consistent with epilepsia partialis continua (EPC), in the above clinical context.

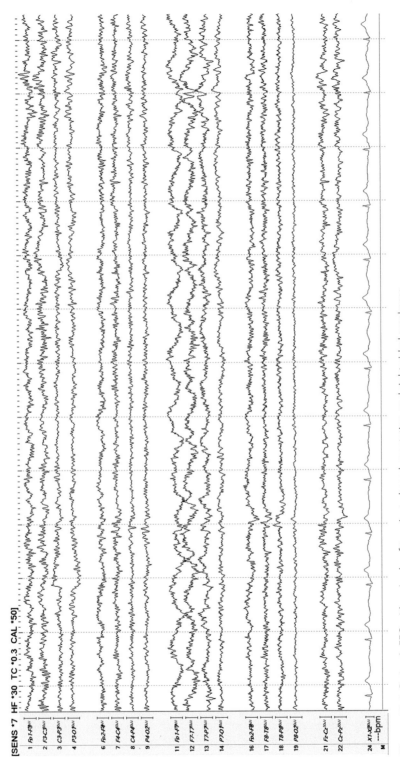

[SENS *7 HF *30 TC *0.3 CAL *50]

1 Fp1-F3
2 F3-C3
3 C3-P3
4 P3-O1

6 Fp2-F4
7 F4-C4
8 C4-P4
9 P4-O2

11 Fp1-F7
12 F7-T7
13 T7-P7
14 P7-O1

16 Fp2-F8
17 F8-T8
18 T8-P8
19 P8-O2

21 Fz-Cz
22 Cz-Pz

24 X1-X2
M ---bpm

Figure 13.4 Patient's EEG with episode of transient altered mentation and right sided weakness.

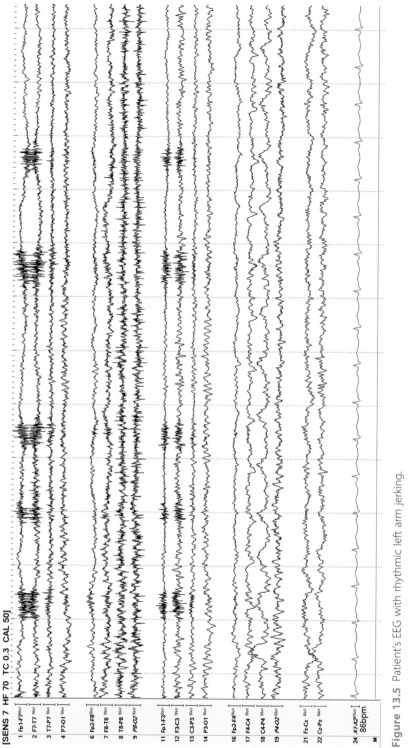

[SENS 7 HF 70 TC 0.3 CAL 50]

1 Fp1-F7 50uV
2 F7-T7 50uV
3 T7-P7 50uV
4 P7-O1 50uV

6 Fp2-F8 50uV
7 F8-T8 50uV
8 T8-P8 50uV
9 P8-O2 50uV

11 Fp1-F3 50uV
12 F3-C3 50uV
13 C3-P3 50uV
14 P3-O1 50uV

16 Fp2-F4 50uV
17 F4-C4 50uV
18 C4-P4 50uV
19 P4-O2 50uV

21 Fz-Cz 50uV
22 Cz-Pz 50uV

24 X1-X2 75uV
86bpm

M

Figure 13.5 Patient's EEG with rhythmic left arm jerking.

Epilepsia Partialis Continua (Kozhevnikov Syndrome)

Epilepsia partialis continua (EPC) is a rare subtype of focal motor status epilepticus, or continuous seizures without impaired awareness. It is characterized by frequent, stereotypical, sometimes arrhythmic jerking movements that most commonly affect the face and limbs and may continue for prolonged periods (sometimes months or years!). EPC may also continue in sleep. Multiple underlying etiologies have been reported including strokes, tumors, brain malformations, and metabolic, infectious, inflammatory, and auto-immune diseases. Rasmussen encephalitis is a rare but severe form of chronic brain inflammation that usually affects a single hemisphere and often presents with EPC. Focal epileptiform activity may correlate with muscle jerking as described earlier. Notoriously resistant to treatment, EPC may continue despite multiple antiseizure medications. Additional treatment with steroids or immunotherapy may be useful depending on the underlying cause [4].

References

1. Britton JW, Frey LC, Hopp JL, et al. Electroencephalography (EEG): An introductory text and atlas of normal and abnormal findings in adults, children, and infants [Internet]. American Epilepsy Society, 2016.
2. Brigo F, Cicero R, Fiaschi A, Bongiovanni LG. The breach rhythm. *Clinical Neurophysiology.* 2011 Nov 1;122(11):2116–20.
3. Gaspard N, Manganas L, Rampal N, Petroff OA, Hirsch LJ. Similarity of lateralized rhythmic delta activity to periodic lateralized epileptiform discharges in critically ill patients. *JAMA Neurology.* 2013 Oct 1;70(10):1288–95.
4. Mameniškienė R, Wolf P. Epilepsia partialis continua: A review. *Seizure.* 2017 Jan 1; 44:74–80.

Chapter **14**

Encephalopathy

Learning Points
- Global cerebral dysfunction
- Generalized rhythmic delta activity (GRDA)
- GPDs with triphasic morphology (triphasic waves)
- Cyclic alternating pattern of encephalopathy (CAPE)

Case A 62-year-old woman with a history of schizophrenia and prior aneurysmal subarachnoid hemorrhage presents to the emergency room after multiple witnessed generalized tonic clonic seizures. She is intubated and sedated upon arrival in the emergency room and an intravenous fosphenytoin load is administered. Figure 14.1 shows a snapshot of her EEG.

How would you describe the EEG findings?
The EEG (Figure 14.1) shows a generalized low voltage background slowing characterized by predominantly low frequency delta slowing and some overriding beta activity.

What is your interpretation?
This "low and slow" recording is typical for encephalopathy.

It is not specific to any etiology. However, medications and/or metabolic abnormalities may be contributors.

Further, excessive beta as noted in this example may also be associated with sedative medications. Reassuringly, there is no evidence of ongoing status epilepticus or seizures during this snapshot of the record.

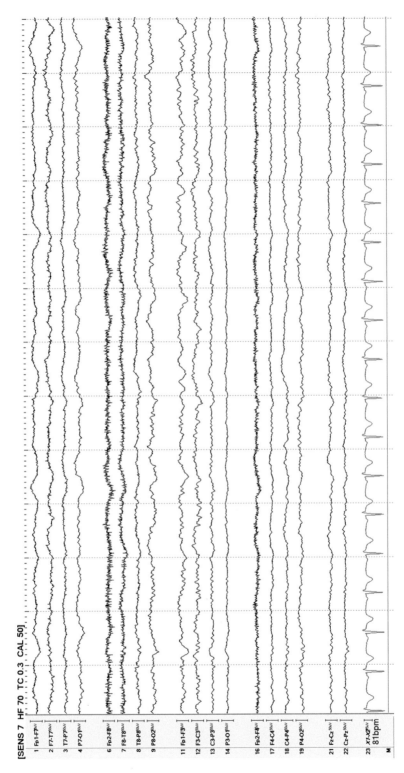

Figure 14.1 Patient's EEG after multiple convulsive seizures.

Global Cerebral Dysfunction

Encephalopathy (global cerebral dysfunction) affects nearly all critically ill individuals with varying degrees of severity, making it a commonly encountered critical care EEG pattern.

Overall, there is a progressive reduction of background voltages (low) and varying amounts of generalized slowing (slow). Eventually, there may be background discontinuity and the posterior dominant rhythm may slow, become less sustained, and eventually be lost entirely. Severe forms may show a loss of EEG reactivity. The electrographic diagnosis and grading of encephalopathy have already been described in Chapter 3. It is important to understand that the EEG patterns of encephalopathy are rarely specific for a particular etiology. However, some patterns may have etiological implications.

The approach to management usually involves correcting the underlying cause(s). In patients with seizures, antiseizure medications and other sedative medications may also contribute to encephalopathy.

Case A 27-year-old man with refractory epilepsy is admitted after an intentional overdose of levetiracetam and zonisamide. Figure 14.2 shows a snapshot of his EEG.

How would you describe the EEG findings?
The EEG (Figure 14.2) shows high amplitude ~1–1.5 Hz generalized rhythmic delta slowing with a frontal predominance.

What is your interpretation?
This pattern is consistent with frontally predominant generalized rhythmic delta activity (GRDA).

Generalized Rhythmic Delta Activity (GRDA)

This is another commonly encountered critical care EEG pattern.

- Most commonly, it is nonspecific to etiology and may occur with several different toxic or metabolic etiologies.
- Less frequently, frontal predominant GRDA (previously called frontal intermittent rhythmic delta activity or FIRDA) may indicate an intracranial mass lesion or raised intracranial pressure.
- Rarely, occipital predominant GRDA (previously called occipital intermittent rhythmic delta activity or OIRDA) may occur with generalized epilepsy disorders (e.g., childhood absence epilepsy).

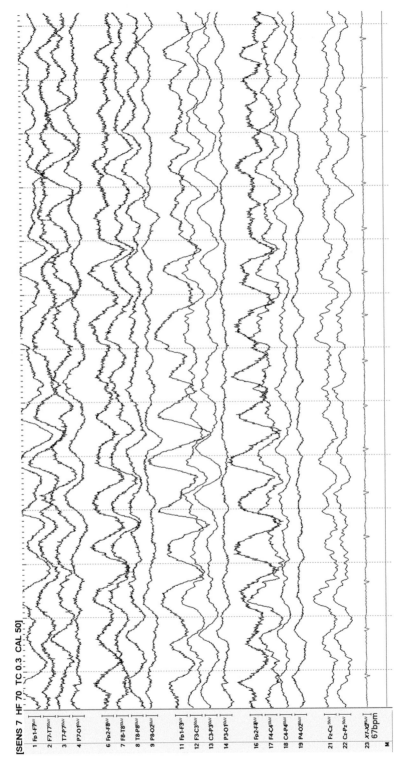

Figure 14.2 Patient's EEG after medication overdose.

Case A 54-year-old man with a history of diabetes mellitus, ischemic heart disease, and chronic renal failure is admitted for an episode of acute on chronic congestive heart failure and deteriorating renal function. Continuous EEG monitoring was requested for persistent somnolence. Figure 14.3 shows a snapshot of his EEG.

How would you describe the EEG findings?
The EEG (Figure 14.3) shows ~1 Hz generalized periodic discharges.

What is your interpretation?
The generalized periodic discharges shown in Figure 14.3 have a distinct "triphasic morphology" (previously called triphasic waves).

What are some typical features of triphasic waves?
Three important features of this pattern include:

- *Triphasic morphology: Each waveform will cross the baseline twice, resulting in three phases with each phase being slightly longer in duration than the previous one. The first is typically directed up (negative), followed by down (positive), and back up again (negative). Sometimes, the first phase may not be as prominent, resulting in a biphasic appearance.*
- *Anterior–posterior (or posterior–anterior) phase lag: Each waveform appears stacked upon another in an anterior–posterior (or posterior–anterior) slant or sliding fashion.*
- *State dependency: Typically, these waveforms are stimulus induced or will emerge during changes of state (arousals).*

Approach to management: This pattern is not usually associated with seizures and therefore antiseizure medications are usually not indicated based on the pattern alone. Treatment involves identifying and addressing the underlying cause(s).

However, if plus terms (+S or +F) are present, the risk of seizures is increased and antiseizure medications may be considered [1,2].

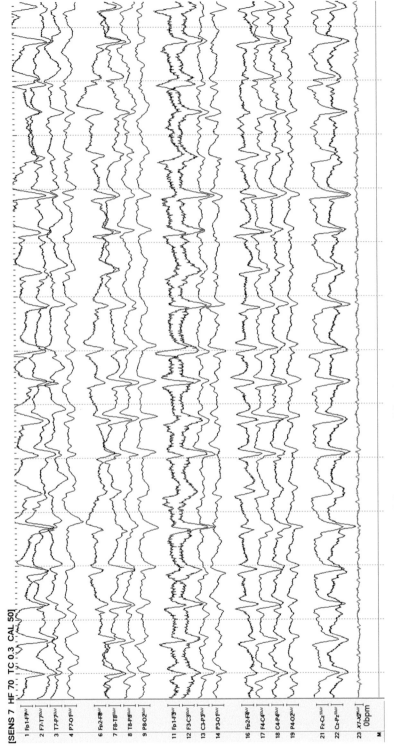

Figure 14.3 Patient's EEG with somnolence and deteriorating renal function.

GPDs with Triphasic Morphology (Triphasic Waves)

This is another distinct pattern seen in critically ill patients.

- Most commonly, triphasic waves occur with several different toxic or metabolic etiologies including hepatic and/or renal dysfunction and medications (see Chapter 4).
- They may also occur with several structural etiologies such as hypoxic ischemic injuries, intracranial hemorrhage, and neurodegenerative disorders including prion diseases.
- Less frequently, generalized periodic discharges with triphasic morphology may actually represent ongoing ictal activity if certain electrographic or clinical criteria are met (seizures or status epilepticus). These so-called ictal triphasic waves are not always distinguishable from typical (nonictal) triphasic waves based on EEG alone as they may lie on the ictal-interictal continuum (IIC). However, a few helpful hints may include:
  - Frequencies ≥ 2.5 Hz
  - Epileptic discharges or [+] terms (+F or +S)
  - Lack of typical features such as phase lag or state dependency.

Approach to management: Most triphasic waves will respond to correction of the underlying cause(s), whenever possible. However, if ictal triphasic waves are suspected, then a trial of antiseizure medications may be indicated (similar to other IIC patterns) with the goal of demonstrating clinical and electrographic improvement with treatment of the electrographic pattern.

If a suspected cause (e.g., a toxic or metabolic etiology) does not completely explain the degree of encephalopathy, or there is a delay in clinical and electrographic improvement despite its correction, then a trial of antiseizure medications should be considered in those with triphasic waves. Intravenous low dose benzodiazepine (e.g., lorazepam) or non-benzodiazepine antiseizure medication (e.g., levetiracetam) may be used to evaluate for a response while on CEEG monitoring.

Trial of low dose lorazepam: Serial small doses (~1 mg each) of lorazepam (total 4 mg) are administered with careful clinical and EEG assessments before and after each dose. Look for resolution of the triphasic waves *and* signs of clinical improvement or appearance of normal electrographic background patterns such as the emergence of a posterior dominant rhythm. Mere suppression of triphasic waves alone does not qualify as success. Most successful responses occur within 2 hours though delayed responses have also been reported. Monitoring of the patient's vital signs is essential given risks of respiratory depression and hypotension with intravenous benzodiazepine use.

Alternatively, if benzodiazepines cannot be safely administered or the response is incomplete, then levetiracetam (or an alternative non-benzodiazepine antiseizure medication) can be given as an intravenous load and maintained for 24–48 hours while observing for a response. Non-benzodiazepine alternatives may show greater response rates, but responses may be delayed [3,4].

Figure 14.4 shows apparent "ictal triphasic waves" in a 68-year-old woman post cardiac arrest and multiple convulsive seizures. Note the ~3 Hz frequency

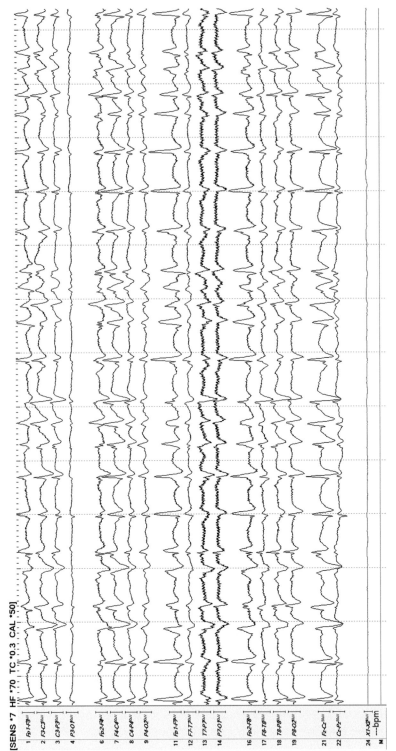

Figure 14.4 "Ictal triphasic waves."

Case A 57-year-old man with suspected meningitis is monitored on CEEG for convulsive episodes. Figures 14.5(a) and (b) show two successive snapshots of his EEG background.

How would you describe the EEG findings?
Figure 14.5(a) shows a pattern of generalized alpha–theta range activity. This appears to alternate with a pattern of generalized rhythmic delta activity as shown in Figure 14.5(b). There is superimposed beta activity throughout.

What is your interpretation?
This pattern of spontaneously alternating background changes is consistent with cyclical alternating pattern of encephalopathy (CAPE).

Of note, these spontaneous alternating cycles of activity may be better appreciated by compressing the recording. For example, Figure 14.5(c) shows a snapshot of the above recording with the time base compressed from the typical 15 seconds to about 3 minutes.

and lack of anterior–posterior phase lag. In this case, despite the pattern's ictal appearance, a trial of levetiracetam was unsuccessful.

Cyclical Alternating Pattern of Encephalopathy (CAPE)
This more recently recognized pattern of encephalopathy refers to two distinct background patterns (including rhythmic and/or periodic patterns) that each last at least 10 seconds and spontaneously alternate with each other regularly for at least six cycles (though they usually continue for much longer).

CAPE may represent a form of state change in encephalopathic patients. Further, some cycles of CAPE may correspond to cycling of other parameters such as respiration, heart rate, blood pressure, motor movements, arousal state, and/or pupillary diameter.

Clinical Significance

- CAPE may represent a favorable prognostic pattern in those with severe encephalopathy and coma depending on the underlying etiology.
- Treatment with antiseizure medication should be avoided given that this pattern may be a manifestation of physiological state changes [5,6].

References
1. Hooshmand H. The clinical significance of frontal intermittent rhythmic delta activity (FIRDA). *Clinical Electroencephalography.* 1983 Jul;14(3):135–7.
2. Lee SI, Kirby D. Absence seizure with generalized rhythmic delta activity. *Epilepsia.* 1988 Jun;29(3):262–7.

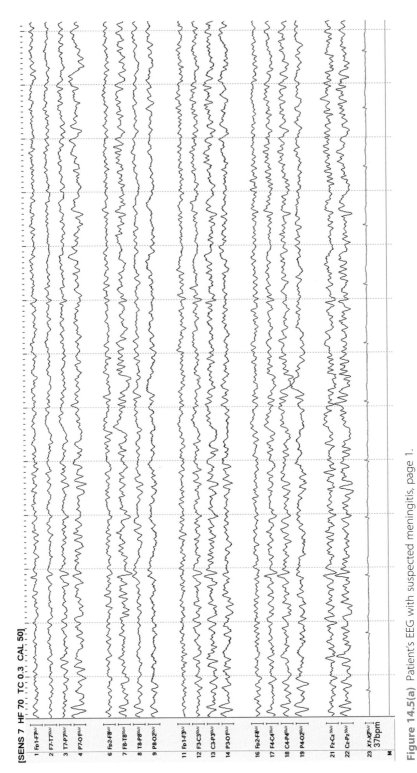

[SENS 7 HF 70 TC 0.3 CAL 50]

1 Fp1-F7⁵⁰ᵘⱽ
2 F7-T7⁵⁰ᵘⱽ
3 T7-P7⁵⁰ᵘⱽ
4 P7-O1⁵⁰ᵘⱽ

6 Fp2-F8⁵ᵘⱽ
7 F8-T8⁵ᵘⱽ
8 T8-P8⁵ᵘⱽ
9 P8-O2⁵⁰ᵘⱽ

11 Fp1-F3⁵ᵘⱽ
12 F3-C3⁵⁰ᵘⱽ
13 C3-P3⁵ᵘⱽ
14 P3-O1⁵⁰ᵘⱽ

16 Fp2-F4⁵ᵘⱽ
17 F4-C4⁵⁰ᵘⱽ
18 C4-P4⁶⁰ᵘⱽ
19 P4-O2⁵⁰ᵘⱽ

21 Fz-Cz⁵⁰ᵘⱽ
22 Cz-Pz⁵⁰ᵘⱽ
23 X1-X2⁵ᵘⱽ
       37bpm
M

Figure 14.5(a) Patient's EEG with suspected meningitis, page 1.

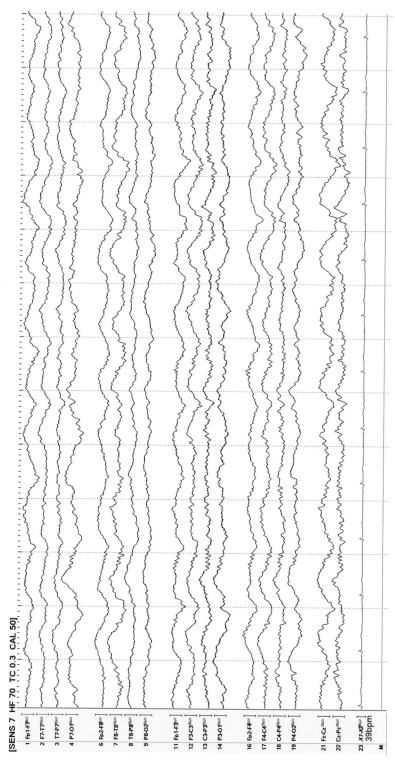

Figure 14.5(b) Patient's EEG with suspected meningitis, page 2.

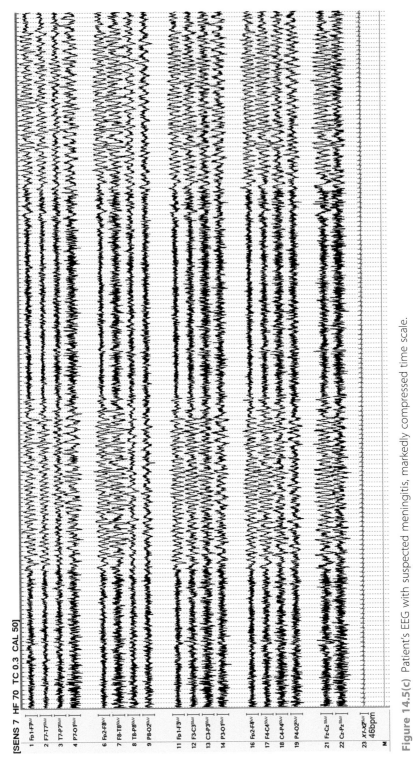

Figure 14.5(c) Patient's EEG with suspected meningitis, markedly compressed time scale.

3. Boulanger JM, Deacon C, Lécuyer D, Gosselin S, Reiher J. Triphasic waves versus nonconvulsive status epilepticus: EEG distinction. *Canadian Journal of Neurological Sciences.* 2006 Jul;33(2):175–80.

4. O'Rourke D, Chen PM, Gaspard N, et al. Response rates to anticonvulsant trials in patients with triphasic-wave EEG patterns of uncertain significance. *Neurocritical Care.* 2016 Apr;24(2):233–9.

5. Hirsch LJ, Fong MW, Leitinger M, et al. American Clinical Neurophysiology Society's Standardized Critical Care EEG Terminology: 2021 version. *Journal of Clinical Neurophysiology.* 2021 Jan 1;38(1):1.

6. Kassab MY, Farooq MU, Diaz-Arrastia R, Van Ness PC. The clinical significance of EEG cyclic alternating pattern during coma. *Journal of Clinical Neurophysiology.* 2007 Dec 1;24(6):425–8.

Chapter

15

Coma

Learning Points
- Extreme delta brush (EDB)

- Alpha-coma and other variants
- Electrocerebral inactivity (ECI)

Case A 24-year-old woman with no prior comorbidities is brought to the emergency room after multiple generalized tonic clonic seizures and personality changes. She is intubated, sedated, and started on IV levetiracetam. Additionally, empiric IV acyclovir is also started for concern of viral encephalitis. Figure 15.1 shows a snapshot of her EEG.

How would you describe the EEG findings?
> *The EEG (Figure 15.1) shows a pattern of generalized rhythmic delta slow waves capped by bursts of low amplitude fast activity over each delta wave.*

What is your interpretation?
> *This pattern of generalized periodic delta slowing with superimposed bursts of fast activity is consistent with extreme delta brush (EDB).*
>
> *In this case, it raises a clinical suspicion for anti-NMDA receptor encephalitis (a type of autoimmune encephalitis).*

Extreme Delta Brush (EDB)

Extreme delta brush refers to a pattern of fast activity (+F) that is superimposed on or associated with rhythmic or periodic delta slowing. It may be generalized (GEDB) or lateralized (LEDB) in appearance.

Clinical Significance

- The pattern is most often associated with anti-NMDA-R encephalitis, though it may not be specific for this condition.

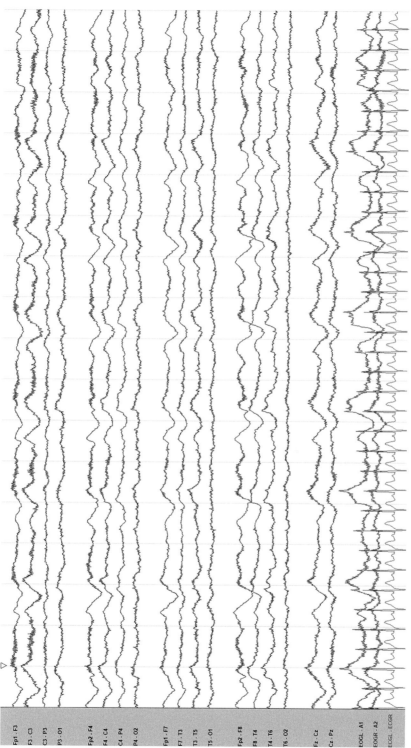

Figure 15.1 Patient's EEG after multiple seizures and subacute personality changes.

- In those with anti-NMDA-R encephalitis, EDB may be associated with poor outcomes including risk of prolonged illness and death. It may also evolve into electrographic status epilepticus.
- Less frequently, it has been reported with other etiologies including temporal lobe epilepsy, hypoxic ischemic brain injury, brain tumors, strokes, and metabolic dysfunction [1–4].

Case A 64-year-old man with hypertension, coronary heart disease, and obstructive sleep apnea presents to the emergency room after an out-of-hospital cardiac arrest followed by return of spontaneous circulation after multiple rounds of cardiopulmonary resuscitation. He is comatose on examination. A snapshot of his EEG is shown in Figure 15.2.

How would you describe the EEG findings?
The EEG (Figure 15.2) shows a pattern of continuous unreactive generalized 6–7 Hz theta activity with a frontal predominance.

What is your interpretation?
In the given clinical context, this pattern of continuous unreactive generalized frontally predominant theta activity may be consistent with theta-coma.

Alpha-Coma and Other Variants

Alpha-coma represents the electroclinical syndrome of clinical coma and corresponding electrographic pattern of generalized alpha activity on EEG, sometimes mimicking wakefulness. Though the electrographic activity may be of alpha frequency (8–13 Hz), its typically continuous, monotonous, and monomorphic appearance with characteristic lack of state dependency or reactivity helps distinguish this pattern from a normal alpha rhythm.

Clinical Significance

- Alpha-coma pattern of hypoxic ischemic brain injury after cardiac arrest may show generalized or frontally predominant unreactive alpha. Sometimes, as in the above case, electrographic activity may be of theta range (alpha–theta or theta-coma).
- Alpha-coma pattern of brainstem etiology (e.g., pontine injury) may show a posterior predominance with some variability or reactivity.

Alpha-coma patterns can be predictive of a poor outcome, depending on the underlying etiology [5,6].

Other Coma Variants

- Spindle coma: shows abundant sleep spindle-like activity.
- Beta-coma: shows continuous diffuse beta activity.

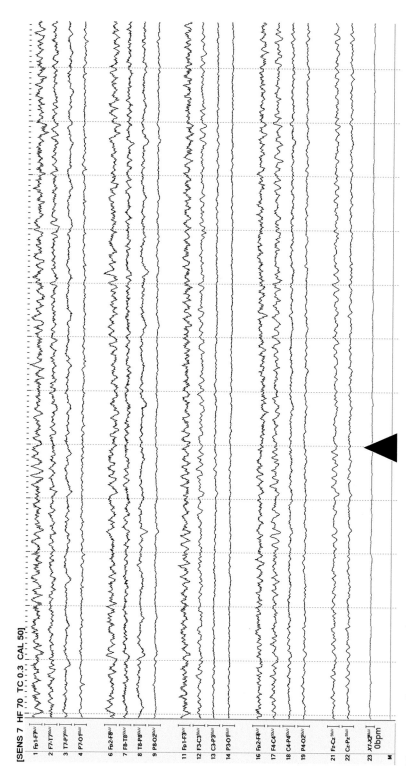

Figure 15.2 Patient's EEG after cardiac arrest. Stimulation is marked with a black arrow.

Case A 68-year-old woman is comatose after an out-of-hospital cardiac arrest. No sign of brainstem activity can be elicited on examination. Figure 15.3 shows a snapshot of her CEEG.

How would you describe the EEG findings?
The EEG (Figure 15.3) shows continuous background suppression without evidence of reactivity or variability.

What is your interpretation?
These findings are consistent with a highly malignant electrographic pattern, post cardiac arrest.

Can this study be used to determine brain death (death by neurological criteria)?
NO. This EEG cannot be used for the purposes of determining brain death as it was not performed using the minimal technical standards for EEG recording in suspected cerebral death as determined by the American Neurophysiology Society (ACNS). A repeat EEG using these criteria should be performed to confirm electrocerebral inactivity (ECI).

Electrocerebral Inactivity (ECI)

The American Clinical Neurophysiology Society defines electrocerebral inactivity as the absence of non-artifactual electrical activity over 2 μV (peak to peak) when recording from scalp electrode pairs 10 or more centimeters apart and compliance with other recording parameters as outlined in its minimal technical standards for EEG recording in suspected cerebral death.

- Brain death is never determined by EEG alone; it is primarily a clinical diagnosis.
- The EEG (using the above criteria) may be included as an ancillary test in brain death protocols.
- Most adults (96.5%) with a clinical diagnosis of brain death show findings of ECI.
- Rarely, electrographic activity may persist in those with severe brainstem injuries, as well as in neonates and children, despite a clinical diagnosis of brain death.

Readers should always refer to their own institutional protocols when brain death is suspected [7–10].

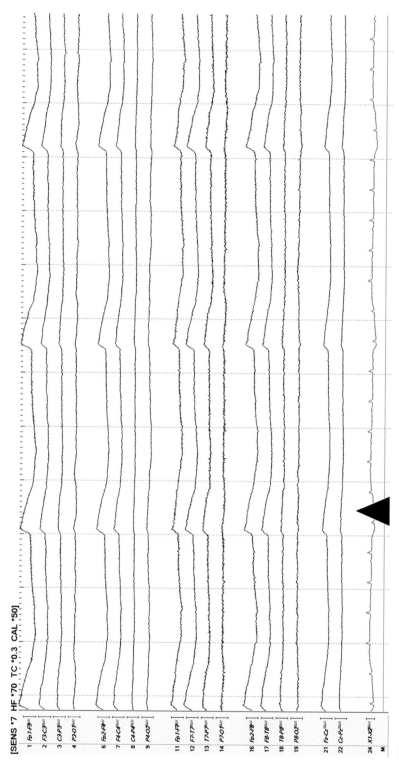

Figure 15.3 Patient's EEG after cardiac arrest. Stimulation is marked with a black arrow.

References

1. Schmitt SE, Pargeon K, Frechette ES, Hirsch LJ, Dalmau J, Friedman D. Extreme delta brush: A unique EEG pattern in adults with anti-NMDA receptor encephalitis. *Neurology*. 2012 Sep 11;79(11):1094–100.
2. Nathoo N, Anderson D, Jirsch J. Extreme delta brush in anti-NMDAR encephalitis correlates with poor functional outcome and death. *Frontiers in Neurology*. 2021;12.
3. Herlopian A, Rosenthal ES, Chu CJ, Cole AJ, Struck AF. Extreme delta brush evolving into status epilepticus in a patient with anti-NMDA encephalitis. *Epilepsy & Behavior Case Reports*. 2017 Jan 1;7:69–71.
4. Hirsch LJ, Fong MW, Leitinger M, et al. American Clinical Neurophysiology Society's Standardized Critical Care EEG Terminology: 2021 version. *Journal of Clinical Neurophysiology*. 2021 Jan 1;38(1):1.
5. Westmoreland BF, Klass DW, Sharbrough FW, Reagan TJ. Alpha-coma: Electroencephalographic, clinical, pathologic, and etiologic correlations. *Archives of Neurology*. 1975 Nov 1;32(11):713–18.
6. Kaplan PW, Genoud D, Ho TW, Jallon P. Etiology, neurologic correlations, and prognosis in alpha coma. *Clinical Neurophysiology*. 1999 Feb 1;110(2):205–13.
7. Fernández-Torre JL, Hernández-Hernández MA, Muñoz-Esteban C. Non confirmatory electroencephalography in patients meeting clinical criteria for brain death: Scenario and impact on organ donation. *Clinical Neurophysiology*. 2013 Dec 1;124(12):2362–7.
8. Nakagawa TA, Ashwal S, Mathur M, Mysore M, Committee for Determination of Brain Death in Infants Children. Guidelines for the determination of brain death in infants and children: An update of the 1987 task force recommendations – executive summary. *Annals of Neurology*. 2012 Apr;71(4):573–85.
9. Machado C, Jeret JS, Shewmon DA, et al. Evidence-based guideline update: Determining brain death in adults: Report of the Quality Standards Subcommittee of the American Academy of Neurology. *Neurology*. 2011 Jan 18;76(3):307–9.
10. Stecker MM, Sabau D, Sullivan LR, et al. American Clinical Neurophysiology Society guideline 6: Minimum technical standards for EEG recording in suspected cerebral death. *The Neurodiagnostic Journal*. 2016 Oct 1;56(4):276–84.

Appendix: Understanding EEG Reports

- Parts of an EEG Report
- Commonly encountered terminology

Currently, there is no universally accepted EEG reporting method, template, or system. The criteria for exactly what should or must be reported vary from source to source. Attempts have been made to standardize EEG reporting, with mixed results. Thus, reports are neither uniform or standardized, sometimes even within a given institution. They still vary widely, from rigid structured reports to freeform dictated prose.

As is the case with other medical reports, these are multipurpose documents: they communicate information to other providers (most of whom are not epileptologists or neurologists), they serve as an objective record of the EEG review that took place (e.g., for medicolegal purposes), and they are submitted for billing and reimbursement purposes.

Some factors influencing what is included in reports and how the information is presented include the specific training and experience of the individual electroencephalographer, as well as "cultural norms" at their medical center. It remains an ongoing challenge to efficiently report all of the potentially clinically useful information while remaining succinct enough for the report to be practical.

Parts of a Typical EEG Report

- **Patient information:** This section contains patient demographic information for identification purposes. It usually contains a brief history or a description of the particular indication for the EEG.
- **Medications:** The EEG report often lists all of the patient's current medications, or sometimes just the clinically relevant medications. This can be useful when determining the effect certain medications may be having on the EEG.
- **Recording conditions, technical description:** This section describes the type of EEG, electrode array, length and timing of recording, and sometimes additional information such as polygraphic channels (EOG, ECG), use of video, use of QEEG, etc.

- **Modulators, activating procedures:** There may or may not be a dedicated section for this, but reports often will described modulating techniques such as hyperventilation, stepped photic stimulation, sleep deprivation, and medication administration/withdrawal.
- **EEG findings:** This is where the heart of the EEG findings usually lies, and again varies widely in terms of the degree of structure, presence of subcategories, etc. Common subcategories include:
  - ○ **EEG background**
  - ○ **Non-epileptiform abnormalities**
  - ○ **Sporadic or interictal epileptiform discharges**
  - ○ **Rhythmic and periodic patterns.**
- **Clinical events:** This is where you may find descriptions of seizures found on the EEG, as well as any other marked or unmarked clinical events.
- **Physiologic patterns, patterns of uncertain significance, and artifacts:** Those reporting EEG (electroencephalographers) vary widely in their tendency to report physiologic patterns, patterns of uncertain clinical significance, or artifacts. Sometimes, they will get their own dedicated category, but often they are included with other background activity.
- **Polygraphic channels:** This is where you will find a description of the single channel cardiac monitor, as well as any other non-EEG channels that may have been added to the recording, such as a limb-EMG channel.
- **Summaries:** Almost all EEG reports contain a summative description of the most pertinent findings of the EEG; however, they will vary in terms of structure (prose vs. bullet points). By convention, many reporters will list the most clinically actionable findings first, and continue in descending order.
- **Interpretations/Clinical significance:** This may or may not be included in the above section, but most EEG reporters will also lay out the basic clinical significance of those findings in the report. *However, importantly, in most cases, EEG recordings cannot specify the particular etiology of a given finding.*

Commonly Encountered EEG Report Terminology

Here we present a table of commonly reported EEG findings, with their respective commonly encountered abbreviations, synonyms, and clinical implications. It is not meant to be comprehensive; it merely presents some of the most commonly encountered terms in acute care EEG reports for reference. When in doubt, *always* discuss individual cases with the reporting electroencephalographer, as many reporters may use any of these terms slightly differently than we have outlined here.

Term	Acronym	Synonyms	Category	Clinical implications
Background disorganization				Potential manifestation of encephalopathy, varying degrees possible
Bilateral independent periodic discharges	BIPDs	**BIPEDs** (bilateral independent periodic epileptiform discharges)	Rhythmic/periodic pattern (RPP)	Two foci of highly irritable cortex seen independently in both hemispheres, indicating elevated seizure risk; this pattern often qualifies for **ictal-interictal continuum (IIC)**
Breach effect		**Breach rhythm**		Focal phenomenon seen with skull defects, craniotomies, etc. Manifest by higher voltages, faster frequencies, and more sharply contoured waveforms
Brief potentially ictal rhythmic discharges	BIRDs	**"Seizure with incomplete evolution"**		Brief seizure-like rhythmic discharges, lasting <10 seconds and without obvious clinical symptoms; these indicate high risk for frank seizures, and may actually represent seizures undetectable on scalp EEG
Burst attenuation				See **Burst suppression**
Burst suppression				Indicating a deep level of encephalopathy; may be medication-induced or can be seen in severe hypoxic ischemic encephalopathy; clinical context is important. This depth of sedation is often used in the treatment of refractory status epilepticus (RSE)

Term	Acronym	Synonyms	Category	Clinical implications
Discontinuity				Periods of intermittent background attenuation of suppression intermixed with cerebral activity; seen in deeper levels of encephalopathy, ranging from mild discontinuity to pronounced **"burst suppression"**
EEG reactivity	EEG-R			Tendency for the EEG pattern to clearly change in frequency or pattern with stimuli; see **"Lack of EEG reactivity"**
Electrocerebral inactivity	ECI			Specific term for the lack of any discernable cerebral activity, only to be used with EEGs performed with brain death protocol
Electroclinical seizure	ECSz		Seizure	Seizure, as diagnosed by a combination of both electrographic and clinical criteria
Electroclinical status epilepticus	ECSE	Often, **non-convulsive status epilepticus**	Status epilepticus	Status epilepticus, as diagnosed by a combination of electrographic findings and clinical response to antiseizure medications
Electrographic seizure	ESz		Seizure	Seizure, as diagnosed purely by electrographic criteria
Electrographic status epilepticus	ESE	Often, **non-convulsive status epilepticus**	Status epilepticus	Status epilepticus, as diagnosed purely by electrographic criteria

Epileptiform discharges, sporadic	Epileptic discharge (Epileptiform discharge)	Can be focal or generalized; EEG transients indicating cortical irritability (alternatively, hyperexcitability) in the specified region, and implying decreased seizure threshold and increased seizure risk; these discharges are not seizures in and of themselves
Excess beta fast activity		Nonspecific finding, most often seen due to medication effects (e.g., benzodiazepines, barbiturates, propofol)
Focal discontinuity		Indicates severe focal cerebral dysfunction; the recording cannot specify the etiology
Focal slowing, continuous		Indicates focal cerebral dysfunction, which could be structural and/or physiologic in nature; the recording cannot specify the etiology
Focal slowing, intermittent		Indicates focal cerebral dysfunction (perhaps subcortical), which could be structural and/or physiologic in nature; the recording cannot specify the etiology
Focal voltage suppression		Indicates severe focal cerebral dysfunction; the recording cannot specify the etiology

215

Term	Acronym	Synonyms	Category	Clinical implications
Generalized periodic discharges	GPDs	**GPEDs** (generalized periodic epileptiform discharges); periodic pattern	Rhythmic/ periodic pattern (RPP)	Generalized cortical irritability, with elevated seizure risk; this pattern often qualifies for **ictal-interictal continuum (IIC)**
Generalized periodic discharges with triphasic morphology	GPDs with triphasic morphology	**Triphasic waves**	Rhythmic/ periodic pattern (RPP)	Classically associated with toxic metabolic encephalopathies, medication effects, and infections; however, this pattern lies on the IIC and can indicate elevated seizure risk and even seizure itself in some circumstances; clinical context is important
Generalized rhythmic delta activity	GRDA	**Generalized rhythmic slowing**; frontal intermittent rhythmic delta activity (**FIRDA**)	Rhythmic/ periodic pattern (RPP)	Nonspecific finding, can be seen with encephalopathy, deep midline subcortical dysfunction, or increased intracranial pressure
Generalized slowing, continuous				Potential manifestation of encephalopathy, varying degrees possible
Generalized slowing, intermittent				Potential manifestation of encephalopathy or drowsiness; clinical context is important

Term	Abbreviation	Synonyms	Category	Description
Generalized spike-wave	GSW	**Generalized sharp-wave, generalized sharp-and-wave, generalized spike-and-wave**	Rhythmic/periodic pattern (RPP)	Generalized cortical irritability; this pattern often qualifies for **ictal-interictal continuum (IIC)**
Generalized voltage suppression				All background EEG activity is <10 μV, indicating a deep level of encephalopathy; may be medication-induced or can be seen in severe hypoxic ischemic encephalopathy; clinical context is important
Ictal-interictal injury continuum	IIC	**Ictal-interictal continuum** (IIC)	Rhythmic/periodic pattern (RPP)	RPPs meeting particular criteria; the concept illustrates that RPPs exist on a continuum between interictal and seizure/status epilepticus itself; a pattern on the ictal-interictal injury continuum does not qualify as a seizure per se, however there is a reasonable chance that it may be contributing to neuronal injury or causing clinical symptoms
Lack of EEG reactivity		Unreactive, lack of reactivity		There is no clear change in EEG frequency or pattern with stimulation; this is an indicator of severe encephalopathy, and is one of many predictors of poor prognosis after cardiac arrest
Lambda waves				Normal finding, positive sharp transients seen in the occipital regions

Term	Acronym	Synonyms	Category	Clinical implications
Lateralized periodic discharges	LPDs	**PLEDs** (periodic lateralized epileptiform discharges)	Rhythmic/ periodic pattern (RPP)	Focal region of highly irritable cortex with elevated seizure risk; this pattern often qualifies for **ictal-interictal continuum (IIC)**
Lateralized rhythmic delta activity	LRDA	**Focal rhythmic slowing**; temporal intermittent rhythmic delta activity (**TIRDA**)	Rhythmic/ periodic pattern (RPP)	Focal region of highly irritable cortex with elevated seizure risk; this pattern often qualifies for **ictal-interictal continuum (IIC)**
Lateralized spike-wave	LSW	Lateralized sharp-wave, lateralized sharp-and-wave, lateralized spike-and-wave	Rhythmic/ periodic pattern (RPP)	Focal region of highly irritable cortex with elevated seizure risk; this pattern often qualifies for **ictal-interictal continuum (IIC)**
Mu rhythm				Normal finding, alpha frequency rhythm seen in the central regions
Multifocal periodic discharges	MfPDs		Rhythmic/ periodic pattern (RPP)	Three or more independent foci of highly irritable cortex, indicating elevated seizure risk; this pattern often qualifies for **ictal-interictal continuum (IIC)**

Term	Abbreviation	Alternative term	Classification	Description
Normal EEG background				Normal study. N.B. A normal EEG does NOT exclude or contradict a clinical diagnosis of seizure or epilepsy!
Paroxysmal clinical events				Broad category including functional seizures and other non-epileptic events
Paroxysmal fast activity	PFA		Epileptiform discharge	See **"Epileptiform discharges, sporadic"**
Posterior dominant rhythm	PDR	**Alpha rhythm**		Often the more prominent feature of the normal awake EEG background
Rhythmic mid-temporal theta of drowsiness	RMTD			Variant of uncertain clinical significance, not known to be associated with epilepsy or increased seizure risk
Sharp transients				A term with variable usage by different EEG reporters, often implying sharp transients without definite epileptiform morphology and some degree of implied uncertainty; discuss with the EEG reporter if the implication is unclear in the report
Sharp waves		**Sharps**	Epileptiform discharge	See **"Epileptiform discharges, sporadic"**
Sharp-slow wave		**Sharp-and-wave, sharp-and-slow wave**	Epileptiform discharge	See **"Epileptiform discharges, sporadic"**

(cont.)

Term	Acronym	Synonyms	Category	Clinical implications
Slowing of the posterior dominant ("alpha") rhythm				Potential manifestation of encephalopathy, varying degrees possible
Spikes			Epileptiform discharge	See **"Epileptiform discharges, sporadic"**
Spike-wave		**Spike-and-wave, spike-wave complex**	Epileptiform discharge	See **"Epileptiform discharges, sporadic"**
Unilateral independent periodic discharges	UIPDs		Rhythmic/ periodic pattern (RPP)	Two foci of highly irritable cortex seen independently within one hemisphere, indicating elevated seizure risk; this pattern often qualifies for **ictal-interictal continuum (IIC)**
Wicket spikes				Variant of uncertain clinical significance, not known to be associated with epilepsy or increased seizure risk

Bibliography

Tatum WO, Olga S, Ochoa JG, et al. American Clinical Neurophysiology Society Guideline 7. *Journal of Clinical Neurophysiology.* 2016;33:328–32.

American Clinical Neurophysiology Society. Guideline Twelve: Guidelines for Long-Term Monitoring for Epilepsy. *Journal of Clinical Neurophysiology.* 2008;25:170–80.

Beniczky S, Aurlien H, Brøgger JC, et al. Standardized Computer-based Organized Reporting of EEG: SCORE. *Epilepsia.* 2013;54:1112–14.

Beniczky S, Aurlien H, Brøgger JC, et al. Standardized Computer-based Organized Reporting of EEG: SCORE – Second version. *Clinical Neurophysiology.* 2017;128:2334–46.

Hirsch LJ, LaRoche SM, Gaspard N, et al. American Clinical Neurophysiology Society's Standardized Critical Care EEG Terminology. *Journal of Clinical Neurophysiology.* 2013;30:1–27.

Index

Printed in the United States
by Baker & Taylor Publisher Services